Controlling and Preventing Errors and Pitfalls in Neonatal Care Delivery

Kim Maryniak

Controlling and Preventing Errors and Pitfalls in Neonatal Care Delivery

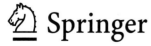 Springer

Kim Maryniak
PhD, RNC-NIC, NEA-BC, Independent Consultant
Casa Grande, AZ, USA

ISBN 978-3-031-25709-4   ISBN 978-3-031-25710-0   (eBook)
https://doi.org/10.1007/978-3-031-25710-0

This Springer imprint is published by the registered company Springer Nature
Switzerland AG
The registered company address is: Gewerbestrasse 11, 6330 Cham, Switzerland

Acknowledgement

Special thanks to our peer reviewers:
Natalie McPherson, BSN, RNC-NIC
Charene Dehne, BSN, RN, EMT-Paramedic, Lt.

Contents

Introduction

Neonates are infants within the first 30 days of life. These patients are one of the most vulnerable populations and require specific knowledge and care. An error that occurs with a neonate has the potential to range from minor to severe, have life-long irreversible consequences, or even be fatal. Nurses have the greatest role in direct patient care, and as members of the most trusted profession have a responsibility to avoid errors and protect these defenseless patients. At this current time, there are global staffing shortages, neonatal patients are sicker and more acute, and there are more task-oriented duties assigned to nurses. These factors can create imbalances and create an overwhelming workload. The aim of *Controlling and Preventing Errors and Pitfalls in Neonatal Care Delivery* is to inform nurses about the most common and the more serious errors made in caring for neonatal patients. This book covers topics about the uniqueness of neonatal patients and common conditions that are seen with patients in the neonatal settings.

This book explores a variety of neonatal conditions, including prematurity, cardiac anomalies, respiratory ailments, gastrointestinal disorders, sepsis, and fluid and electrolyte imbalances. Causes, signs, and management of these conditions are discussed. The types of errors, consequences, detection, and monitoring for nursing errors are included. There are multiple types of errors that can occur during the care of neonatal patients related to handling, assessment, and treatment. Medication errors can also occur which can have detrimental consequences. Multiple negative outcomes can arise from nursing errors, affecting the patient, family, and even the healthcare professionals involved. Negative effects at an organization-wide level may also occur as a result of errors.

There are a variety of strategies that can be implemented to detect and monitor for nursing errors. Process improvement and quality assurance through use of effective tools can assist with detection and monitoring of errors. System tactics and effective communication are also vital to make improvements. A workplace culture that is supportive with effective leadership can also assist in reduction of errors.

Application of just culture is discussed, and how that framework can be used to determine cause of errors, as well as the potential need for system and process improvements. Predisposing and contributing factors for nursing errors will be reviewed, which can include personal factors, such as health or knowledge, processes, and environmental factors. Often a combination of factors can exist, which can create a higher risk for errors.

The book describes how errors can be avoided with necessary precautions and managed appropriately based on current evidence-based practice. There are many practices that have been identified in studies to help prevent nursing errors, such as the use of bundles to prevent hospital-acquired conditions. System and personal considerations can also prevent nursing errors.

Case studies and examples are provided, demonstrating effective practices for reducing patient errors with neonatal patients. Recommendations for further study are also provided.

Overview of Common Conditions in Neonatal Settings

Transition to Extrauterine Life Complications

Fetal circulation and neonatal circulation are very different, and several events need to occur for a successful transition to extrauterine life. The placenta is essential for the fetus as the source of gas exchange, metabolic processes, and excretion. Oxygenated blood is carried from the placenta to the fetus, with a minimal amount of blood flowing to the lungs, which are not yet in use. The inferior vena cava enters the right atrium and most of the blood from the right atrium moves across the foramen ovale into the left atrium. The blood in the left atrium has good oxygenation and passes to the left ventricle and the ascending aorta. The majority of the blood is sent to the brain and heart via the aorta, while blood returns from the head and upper extremities and returns to the right atrium through the superior vena cava. Carbon dioxide and other wastes are carried from the fetus to the placenta through the two umbilical arteries.

Fetal circulation is maintained by a low vascular resistance from the placenta, a high vascular resistance from the lungs, and the presence of vessels and openings to allow shunting of blood. The foramen ovale allows blood to move from the right atrium to the left atrium. The ductus venosus shunts some of the left umbilical vein blood flow into the inferior vena cava, which allows oxy-

K. Maryniak, *Controlling and Preventing Errors and Pitfalls in Neonatal Care Delivery*, https://doi.org/10.1007/978-3-031-25710-0_1

genated blood from the placenta to bypass the liver. The ductus arteriosus connects the pulmonary artery to the proximal descending aorta. In utero, the fetus makes breathing movements but the lungs are not functional for breathing. There is lung fluid present, and there is a high vascular resistance from constricted blood vessels within the lungs. The fetus has low systemic vascular resistance and high pulmonary vascular resistance (Verklan et al. 2020).

At birth, changes must occur rapidly. Systemic vascular resistance is increased when the cord is clamped, and pulmonary vascular resistance is decreased with lung expansion. Oxygen is critical for the dilation of blood vessels, so lung fluid in the airways and alveoli must be expelled before the first breath to provide effective air exchange. Most of the fluid is squeezed out when the neonate progresses through the birth canal and the rest is absorbed into the lung tissue, being replaced by air with the first breath, which also increases pulmonary blood flow (Verklan et al. 2020).

There is a functional closure of the foramen ovale within the first 24 h of life from the decreased pulmonary vascular resistance, increased pulmonary blood volume, and increasing pressure in the left atrium. The foramen ovale may take years to close anatomically. The ductus venosus also functionally closes at birth and closes anatomically at 1–2 weeks. The umbilical cord clamping decreases blood flow through the ductus venosus and increases systemic vascular resistance and blood flow to the liver. Closure of the ductus arteriosus also occurs functionally within the first 24 h and closes anatomically within the first 2 weeks. An initial increase in oxygen at birth will constrict the ductus. When the placenta is removed, prostaglandin E2 (PGE), which maintains the vasodilatation of the ductus, and other vasoactive substances are decreased, and there is an increase in pulmonary blood flow. This further constricts and closes the ductus arteriosus. The first breath occurs due to multiple factors such as a continuation of fetal breathing, chemical factors, sensory stimulation, and chest recoil. Continued breathing assists in lung adaptation of fetal lung fluid to oxygen (Verklan et al. 2020).

There can be difficulties in the transition to extrauterine life which can cause complications. The evidence shows that most neonates in the United States are born vigorously, with only 10% of neonates needing some form of assistance, and less than 1% requiring intensive resuscitation. Every delivery requires one person whose only responsibility is the care of the newborn to start resuscitation, including positive-pressure ventilation and chest compressions. Other individuals who can perform a complete resuscitation must be immediately available (American Academy of Pediatrics and American Heart Association 2021).

The first breath may be problematic from opposing surface tension and lung fluid viscosity. There is also an increase in surface tension when there is little or no surfactant. Primary apnea occurs when, in utero, there are increased respirations due to asphyxiation. The neonate becomes apneic and then bradycardic with a slight increase in blood pressure. At birth, management is needed with stimulation and oxygen. Secondary apnea happens when asphyxia continues beyond primary apnea, with gasping, bradycardia, and hypotension. Stimulation and oxygen will not manage secondary apnea, and treatment consists of immediate resuscitation. If there is not a rapid transition of the lungs to become the site for gas exchange, then cyanosis, hypoxia, and bradycardia quickly occur. There are also complications that interfere with opening pulmonary vasculature, such as hyperviscous blood, persistent pulmonary hypertension (PPHN), poor or no surfactant, and asphyxia. There may also be failures of vessel closures, such as patent ductus arteriosus, which creates persistent fetal circulation (American Academy of Pediatrics and American Heart Association 2021; Verklan et al. 2020). Further discussion of cardiac problems will be provided in later sections.

Persistent pulmonary hypertension of the newborn (PPHN) occurs when there is elevated pulmonary vascular resistance and systemic arterial hypoxemia, most often associated with perinatal asphyxia. PPHN is associated with hypoglycemia, hypocalcemia, hyperviscosity syndrome, sepsis, term and post-term. Risk factors for PPHN are intrauterine closure of the ductus, abnormal responsiveness of the pulmonary vasculature to hypoxia, repeated intrauterine hypoxia, regional alveolar hypoxia, congenital diaphragmatic hernia, pulmonary hypoplasia, alterations in vaso-active mediator levels, microthrombus formation in the pulmonary vascular bed, and meconium aspiration syndrome. Signs of PPHN may include cyanosis, respiratory distress, tachypnea, difference in preductal and post-ductal arterial circulation, and hypotension. PPHN management may include inotropes, low stimulus, sedation, paralytics, maintaining hemoglobin and fluid and electrolytes, nitrous oxide, and ECMO (Gardner et al. 2020; Verklan et al. 2020).

Perinatal asphyxia can occur during the perinatal period which severely reduces oxygen delivery and can lead to acidosis and organ failure. Asphyxia is usually caused by placental insufficiency but may also occur with hypoplastic lungs, premature lungs, pulmonary masses, cardiac defects that compromise circulation, or neurological hemorrhages that can cause hypoxia. Risk factors for perinatal asphyxia include maternal hypertension, intrauterine growth restriction (IUGR), placental abruption, fetal anemia, post-maturity, and induction of labor. Signs of asphyxia include depressed cardiopulmonary and neurological responsiveness, low APGAR scores, hyaline membrane disease or intracranial bleed with premature neonates, or meconium or persistent pulmonary hypertension with post-term neonates. Management of perinatal asphyxia includes treatment of the underlying cause, such as maternal medications or condition, acute blood loss, or neurological, cardiac or neurological malformations (Verklan et al. 2020).

Preterm and Post-term

Gestational age is assessed by using a maturity rating and classification tool and should be performed as soon as possible after birth. With the tool, each component is assessed and scored by comparing observations of the neonate with the visual depictions on tool. The components related to neuromuscular maturity are posture, square window, arm recoil, popliteal angle, scarf sign, and heel to ear. The components that are included in the physical maturity include skin, lanugo, plantar surface, breast, eye/ear, and genitals. Each component is scored and the total provides the maturity rating score. The maturity rating score will give an estimated gestational age (Rogelet and Brorsen 2016; Verklan et al. 2020). A link to an assessment tool is found in the Resources section of this chapter.

A term neonate is one who is between 37- and 42 weeks gestation. They have an average weight and certain characteristics. Physical characteristics of a term neonate are a flexed posture, a full range of motion, smooth skin, vernix present in body creases, some lanugo, soft fontanels, pliable cartilage of ears, plantar creases on the whole sole of foot, breast tissue, and labia majora covering the minora for females or rugae on scrotum for males (Rogelet and Brorsen 2016; Verklan et al. 2020).

A preterm neonate is one who is less than 37 weeks gestation. Physical characteristics of a preterm neonate include loos or transparent skin, visible, and superficial veins on the abdomen and scalp, lack of subcutaneous fat, lanugo covering most of the body, abundant vernix, short-appearing extremities, few creases on soles of feet, protruding abdomen, short nails, small genitalia, labia majora may be open for females, rare rugae is found in males, and poor muscle tone. A preterm neonate has a high risk for multiple complications. These complications can include respiratory distress, hypoxia, apnea, immature central nervous and gastrointestinal systems, temperature instability, feeding difficulties, necrotizing enterocolitis, hypoglycemia, infection and sepsis, hyperbilirubinemia, intraventricular hemorrhage, anemia, polycythemia, patent ductus arteriosus, and retinopathy of prematurity (Rogelet and Brorsen 2016; Verklan et al. 2020).

A post-term neonate is one who is greater than 42 weeks gestation. Characteristics of a post-term neonate are dry and flaky skin, long fingernails, abundant scalp hair, depleted subcutaneous fat and skin sagginess, lack of vernix and lanugo, and may have a wide-eyed appearance. A post-term neonate also has a high risk for associated complications, such as stillbirth, meconium aspiration, respiratory distress, hypoxia, macrosomia, birth trauma, hypoglycemia, and seizures (Rogelet and Brorsen 2016; Verklan et al. 2020).

Birthweight and Growth

Neonates born at lower birthweights are more susceptible to issues. Very low birthweight (VLBW) neonates are those who are born at a weight less than 1500 g. These neonates have additional vulnerabilities and higher morbidity and mortality related to physiological prematurity. This means that even minor changes can have major effects on physiology. VLBW neonates are at higher risk for developing necrotizing enterocolitis (NEC), retinopathy of prematurity (ROP), hearing impairment, intraventricular hemorrhage (IVH), periventricular leukomalacia (PVL), infection, cerebral palsy, and cognitive delays (Gleason and Juul 2018; Lee et al. 2020).

Extremely low birthweight (ELBW) neonates are defined as those weighing less than 1000 g, and are usually associated with younger gestations. ELBW neonates are especially vulnerable due to extreme physiological prematurity. For these neonates, even minute changes can have large effects. ELBW neonates are at risk for the same morbidities as VLBW neonates as well as others. The most common morbidity associated with ELBW neonates is chronic lung disease. Other conditions include patent ductus arteriosus (PDA), congenital heart disease (CHD), sepsis, shock, air leak syndromes, pain, profound hearing impairment, and increased risk of blindness. Evidence shows that a standardized approach to providing care for VLBW and ELBW neonates has been the most successful (Gleason and Juul 2018; Lee et al. 2020).

Growth charts examine size measurements in relation to gestation. The components of growth chart are length, head circumference, and weight. Assessment of neonatal growth can determine potential issues by comparing with normal standards. A neonate who is average for gestational age (AGA) is plotted between the 10th and 90th percentiles on the growth chart (see Fig. 1.1).

Small for gestational age (SGA) neonates are less than 10th percentile on growth charts. SGA neonates have distinctive characteristics, such as a large head compared to the body, skin that is loose and dry, scant scalp hair, decreased subcutaneous fat, emaciated appearance, depressed abdomen, sunken anterior fontanel,

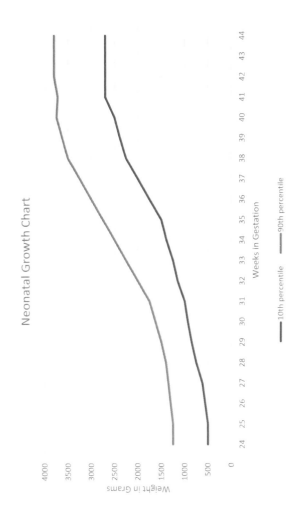

Fig. 1.1 Neonatal growth chart example

vigorous cry, and irritability. SGA can be caused by maternal, intrauterine, and fetal factors. Maternal factors include hypertension, chronic kidney disease, diabetes, cardiac or respiratory disease, malnutrition, blood disorders, infection, and substance use. Intrauterine factors are decreased uterine or placental blood flow, abruptio placentae, placenta previa, and chorioamnionitis. Fetal factors include multiple gestation, infection, birth defects, and chromosomal abnormalities. SGA neonates are at higher risk for some disorders, such as hypoglycemia, cold stress, polycythemia, respiratory distress, and temperature instability (Rogelet and Brorsen 2016; Verklan et al. 2020).

Large for gestational age (LGA) neonates are those who are greater than 90th percentile on growth charts. LGA is typically caused by genetics, maternal weight gain, or maternal diabetes. There are risks associated with LGA, including prolonged or difficult vaginal delivery, increased risk of Cesarean section, birth trauma, hypoglycemia, polycythemia, increased incidence of birth defects, respiratory distress, and hyperbilirubinemia (Rogelet and Brorsen 2016; Verklan et al. 2020).

Infections and Sepsis

Infections are commonly seen in neonates due to their susceptibility to immature protective mechanisms, higher chances of breeches in the line of defense from invasive procedures, and contact with potential contaminants from the vagina and the environment. There are also multiple risk factors for developing infections in the neonate, including maternal, neonatal, and other factors. Maternal risk factors are premature labor, fever, urinary tract infection, chorioamnionitis, group B strep positive or unknown status, premature or prolonged rupture of membranes, prolonged or difficult labor, poor prenatal care, lower socioeconomic status, inadequate nutrition, multiple pregnancies, and substance abuse. Neonatal risk factors are congenital anomalies, fetal distress, asphyxia, meconium aspiration, prematurity, VLBW and ELBW, and inborn errors of metabolism. Other risk factors for infection are resuscitation, invasive procedures, length of hospitalization, use of anti-infective medications, delayed enteral feedings, and total parenteral nutrition (Verklan et al. 2020).

The cause of sepsis is the spread of invading organisms and any byproducts through the bloodstream and tissues. These organisms can be bacterial, viral, fungal, or parasitic organisms. Early-onset sepsis occurs within the first 72 h of life from maternal transmission during pregnancy or delivery, or immediately following delivery, with group B strep being the most common cause. Late-onset sepsis happens after 72 h of age as a result of community-acquired or healthcare-associated infections. Congenital viral infections are classified using the TORCH acronym: T—Toxoplasmosis, O—Other (syphilis, varicella, parvovirus, human immunodeficiency virus, enterovirus), R—Rubella, C—Cytomegalovirus (CMV), and H—Herpes simplex (Verklan et al. 2020).

General signs of infections and sepsis are seen in the early and late stages. Early signs include apnea, tachypnea, increased oxygen requirements, tachycardia, widened pulse pressure, flushing, full pulses, lethargy, hypotonia, temperature instability, behavioral changes, feeding intolerance, metabolic acidosis, glucose instability, either increased or decreased total white blood cells, an increased immature to total (I:T) white blood cell ratio, and thrombocytopenia. Signs in the late stage are decreased systolic pressure, narrowing of pulse pressure, renal failure, splenomegaly, hepatomegaly, seizures, multiple organ dysfunction syndrome, lactic acidosis, higher blood urea nitrogen (BUN) and creatinine, and hyperbilirubinemia. Management of infections and sepsis depends on the causative organism, stage of the infection, and comorbidities. Anti-infectives are given based on the invading organism. Other support strategies are maintenance of a neutral thermal environment, isolation, fluid and electrolyte balance, adequate oxygenation and ventilation, supporting perfusion, removal of central lines, exchange transfusion, and administration of intravenous immunoglobulin (IVIG) (Verklan et al. 2020).

Fluid, Electrolyte, and Glucose Imbalances

Fluid and electrolyte imbalances are common in the neonatal population. A term neonate has about 80% body water content, and a premature neonate can have up to 85–90% body water content. Additionally, there is a relatively large surface area with neonates, which increases with decreasing size. This combination of factors creates increased fluid requirements with neonates. Fluids and electrolytes are also influeced by neonatal factors such as a limited ability to concentrate urine, have high metabolic rates, inefficient kidneys, intrapartum stress can delay a neonate's voiding, there is a 10–15% weight loss in the first week of life, and there are increased insensible water losses with VLBW, ELBW, and extreme prematurity (Kenner et al. 2019).

Water is distributed both inside and outside of cells. The area within a cell is called intracellular, where the majority of the total body water is located. Extracellular locations include intravascular (within the blood vessel) and interstitial (the area between and around the cells). Fluid can be lost through sensible, insensible, and abnormal losses. Sensible losses include fluid loss through urine, stool, and sweat, while insensible losses those occurring through the skin and lungs. Abnormal losses occur with conditions such as diarrhea, ostomy drainage, wounds, aspirates, blood loss, chest tube drainage, and gastrointestinal anomalies such as gastroschisis and omphalocele. Other factors that can increase fluid loss are phototherapy, use of non-humidified air or oxygen, increased respiratory rate and effort, increased activity, radiant heat, cold stress and hypothermia, and conditions that cause further increases in metabolic rate (Kenner et al. 2019).

Neonatal edema can be caused by a variety of factors, including over-administration of fluid, pathological conditions, medications, and renal failure. Conditions related to edema are congenital heart defects, respiratory distress syndrome, asphyxia, sepsis, hydrops fetalis, and syndrome of inappropriate antidiuretic hormone secretion (SIADH). Signs of neonatal edema are weight gain, tachycardia, increased or decreased urine output, overload of intravascular volume, opening or enlarging of patent ductus arteriosus (PDA), and pulmonary edema (Kenner et al. 2019).

Neonatal dehydration may be caused by various factors, including under-administration of fluid, poor feeding, and electrolyte imbalances such as hypernatremia and hyperglycemia. Signs of neonatal dehydration are lethargy, irritability, poor skin turgor, sunken fontanels, and decreased urinary output (Kenner et al. 2019).

An important electrolyte is sodium, which is a major component of extracellular fluid. Sodium takes part in the regulation of acid–base balance, tissue osmolality, enzyme activity, and is essential for the retention of body water. Hypernatremia is an elevated sodium level, caused by dehydration, over-administration of sodium supplementation, osmotic changes, and diuresis. Signs of hypernatremia are irritability, lethargy, vomiting, and seizures. Hyponatremia is a decreased sodium level from overhydration, water retention, and hypovolemia. Hyponatremia signs include vomiting, lethargy, poor perfusion, edema, and seizures. Management of sodium imbalances is based on treating the underlying cause(s). In hyponatremia, sodium replacement needs to be done slowly (Kenner et al. 2019).

Potassium is a major component of intracellular fluid, which participates in enzyme activity, central nervous system function, regulation of tissue osmolality, glycogen use, and cardiac function. Potassium values may be falsely elevated by hemolysis of blood samples. Hyperkalemia is an elevated potassium level, caused by acidosis, renal failure, trauma, bruising, and bleeding. Signs of hyperkalemia may include electrocardiogram (ECG) changes such as a widened QRS complex, peaked T-waves, lengthening of PR interval, unclear P wave, and ventricular fibrillation. Other hyperkalemia signs include decreased urine output, lethargy, and decreased muscle tone. Management of hyperkalemia may include administration of polystyrene sulfonates, calcium, and insulin with glucose drip. Hypokalemia is a decreased potassium level, caused by potassium losses through the gastrointestinal tract, decreased potassium intake, and renal losses.

Signs of hypokalemia may include ECG changes, such as a shortened ST segment, flattened or inverted T-waves, and appearance of a "U" wave. Other hypokalemia signs include intestinal ileus and gastric dilation. Management of hypokalemia is to correct any acid–base or other electrolyte imbalances, use potassium-sparing diuretics, and potassium supplementation (which must be given slowly) (Kenner et al. 2019).

Calcium is a component of the extracellular fluids (ECF), and is essential in blood coagulation and neuromuscular function. Hypocalcemia is a decreased calcium level caused by asphyxia, prematurity, stressors, maternal diabetes, hypoparathyroidism, vitamin D metabolism defects, and phosphate imbalance. Signs of hypocalcemia include irritability, muscle twitches, jitteriness, tremors, poor feeding, lethargy, and seizures. Management of hypocalcemia includes treatment of the underlying cause, and calcium supplements may be needed (Kenner et al. 2019).

Neonatal energy requirements should focus on growth, and the majority of energy is supplied as glucose as the main carbohydrate. Insulin and glucagon are important hormones that control the glucsoe metabolism.

Hypoglycemia is determined based on multiple factors in the neonate, including post-birth age in the first 48 h of life, gestational age, if the neonate is symptomatic, and presence of acute illness. Hypoglycemia may be caused by hyperinsulinemia, decreased production or glucose availability, increased glucose utilization, endocrine abnormalities, or other conditions. Hypoglycemia caused by hyperinsulinemia is seen with maternal diabetes, neonatal hemolytic disease, Beckwith–Wiedemann syndrome, islet cell hyperplasia, exchange transfusion, maternal tocolytic agents, LGA, abrupt discontinuation of intravenous glucose, and insulin-producing tumors. Decreased production or availability of glucose is found with intrauterine growth retardation (IUGR), metabolism defects, prematurity, difficult or delayed feedings, and no oral or peripheral glucose supplementation. Increased glucose utilization is found with cold stress, sepsis, respiratory distress, and perinatal asphyxia. Endocrine abnormalities that cause hypoglycemia include adrenal insufficiency, pan-hypopituitarism, hypothyroidism, and glucagon or epinephrine deficiency. Other conditions related to hypoglycemia are polycythemia, central nervous system abnormalities, congenital heart disease, and maternal use of beta-blockers. The signs of neonatal hypoglycemia may include jitteriness, irritability, lethargy, hypotonia, apnea, cyanosis, weak or high-pitched cry, poor feeding, vomiting, seizures, and coma. Management strategies may include dextrose administration, oral feedings, glucagon, and steroids (Kenner et al. 2019).

Hyperglycemia is caused by infusions with dextrose included, certain medications, sepsis, hypoxia, surgery, pancreatic lesions, hyperosmolar formula, physiologic stress, and immature glucose transport proteins. Signs of hyperglycemia are non-specific and may include dehydration, irritability, and other electrolyte imbalances. Management of hyperglycemia includes reducing dextrose concentrations, changing from intravenous (IV) to oral feeding if able, frequent glucose monitoring, and intravenous insulin (Kenner et al. 2019).

Blood Disorders

There are common blood disorders that can be seen in neonatal patients. In the neonate, anemia can occur from a variety of causes. Anemia of prematurity is seen in preterm neonates, where the red blood cell mass is decreased at birth but hemoglobin is stable. The survival of red blood cells is shorter in premature neonates. Blood loss, whether fetal, maternal, or neonatal, causes a drop in hematocrit and reticulocytes, resulting in anemia. Anemia can also be caused by hemolysis, hereditary disorders, and decreased red blood cell production. Diagnosis of anemia is made through blood tests as well as history and physical examination. Anemia, particularly through acute blood loss, can cause acidosis, shock, or poor perfusion. Signs of anemia include pallor, respiratory distress, jaundice, and hepatosplenomegaly. Anemia management is individualized, depending on severity, risk factors, and comorbidities. Management for healthy neonates is usually observed to see if the body will correct it. Other management may include recombinant erythropoietin (EPO), iron, and/or transfusion. Indications for transfusion include significant respiratory or congenital heart disease, ABO incompatibility, hematocrit less than 31%, or severe signs such as increasing oxygen needs, apneic episodes, sustained tachycardia, and poor weight gain (Rogelet and Brorsen 2016; Verklan et al. 2020).

Neonatal bleeding can occur from several conditions, such as transitory deficiency in clotting factors and disturbances of clotting associated with diseases, and interventions. Transitory deficiency in clotting factors may be a result of total parenteral nutrition or antibiotics that lack vitamin K in premature neonates. Maternal medications can also cause bleeding in the first 24 h, such as phenytoin, phenobarbital, coumadin, or salicylates, which interfere with vitamin K effects or synthesis. Clotting disturbances can be seen with inherited abnormalities, necrotizing enterocolitis (NEC), disseminated intravascular coagulation (DIC), infection, or shock. Interventions such as extracorporeal membrane oxygenation (ECMO) are also associated with bleeding. Platelet disorders can also cause bleeding. Assessment includes findings that are suspicious for bleeding, such as petechiae, superficial ecchymosis, mucosal bleeding, an enlarged spleen, jaundice, and abnormal retinal findings. Management of bleeding is individualized and is based on the underlying cause as well as the level of illness of the neonate. Types of management include transfusion with blood or blood products, use of vitamin K, clotting factor concentrates, or cryoprecipitate (Gardner et al. 2020; Verklan et al. 2020).

Thrombocytopenia in the neonate is a platelet count of less than 150,000/mcL, and can be a common finding with ill neonates. Thrombocytopenia may be caused by alloimmune or autoimmune disorders, placental insufficiency, perinatal asphyxia, congenital or other infections, NEC, or medications. Thrombocytopenia is diagnosed through laboratory testing, history, and assessment. Signs of thrombocytopenia are petechiae or bruising, hepatosplenomegaly, jaundice, limb enlargement, or hemangioma. Thrombocytopenia is managed based on the underlying cause. Platelet transfusions may be indicated with bleeding or platelet counts of less than 20,000/mcL, with or without steroids (Gardner et al. 2020; Verklan et al. 2020).

Neonatal polycythemia is a hematocrit level of greater than 65% in venous samples or 63% in arterial samples. Polycythemia causes blood to become hyperviscous, which decreases oxygen transport to tissues. Hypoxia and acidosis create more viscosity, decreased plasma glucose, higher risk for formation of microemboli, and significant damage to organs. Polycythemia may be caused by a variety of conditions, such as delayed cord clamping, cord stripping, holding baby below mother at delivery, maternal-to-fetal transfusion, twin-to-twin transfusion, forceful uterine contraction before cord clamping, placental insufficiency, maternal diabetes, congenital adrenal hyperplasia, maternal medications, dehydration, and certain syndromes or trisomies. Signs of polycythemia may include poor feeding, lethargy, hypotonia, apnea, tremors, jitteriness, seizures, cerebral thrombosis, cyanosis, tachypnea, heart murmurs, congestive heart failure, cardiomegaly, increased pulmonary resistance, decreased glomerular filtration, low sodium excretion, renal vein thrombosis, hematuria, proteinuria, thrombosis, thrombocytopenia, jaundice, persistent hypoglycemia, hypocalcemia, testicular infarcts, NEC, and DIC. Polycythemia is managed based on condition and cause. An increase of fluids and exchange transfusion may be warranted (Gardner et al. 2020; Verklan et al. 2020).

Neutropenia occurs with an absolute neutrophil count (ANC) of less than 1000 mcL. Neutropenia can be caused by decreased neutrophil production, increased neutrophil destruction, idiopathic neutropenia of prematurity, drug-induced neutropenia, and pseudoneutropenia. Management of neutropenia is based on the underlying causes and may include the use of stimulating factors, antibiotics if infection is suspected, or even bone marrow biopsy (Gardner et al. 2020; Verklan et al. 2020).

When a Rh-negative mother is exposed to foreign antigens, such as with a Rh-positive fetus, there can be a maternal–fetal blood Rh incompatibility. Without treatment, Rh-negative mothers are at risk for fetal demise or delivering a neonate with hydrops fetalis. Many neonates will need only minor treatments such as phototherapy for jaundice. Other neonates will be severely affected, such as those with profound anemia, ongoing hemolysis, enlarged liver and spleen, high white blood count, and thrombocytopenia. Prevention is vital with potential Rh incompatibility, including avoiding maternal exposure to unnecessary medical procedures such as transfusions and amniocentesis. Administration of Rho (D) immune globulin should be given to unsensitized Rh-negative mothers at 28 weeks gestation and within 72 h after giving birth. Use of the immunoglobulin prophylactically should also be done following abortion, amniocentesis, chorionic villi sampling, and transplacental hemorrhage. Hydrops fetalis, or fetal hydrops, is a condition of abnormal collections of fluid. Immune hydrops fetalis is caused by severe Rh incompatibility. Hydrops fetalis may present with ascites, edema, pericardial effusion, and pleural effusion, and can be associated with placental edema or polyhydramnios. Hydrops is usually seen on prenatal ultrasound if there are significant accumulations of fluid. The condition is associated with high morbidity and mortality (Gardner et al. 2020; Verklan et al. 2020).

Type O mothers who have A or B antigens will attack type A or B blood cells in the fetus, which is known as ABO hemolytic disease. ABO hemolytic disease is a common cause of red blood cell (RBC) hemolysis and hyperbilirubinemia. Many cases occur in firstborns, and most neonates will have mild to moderate signs. Hyperbilirubinemia will present in the first 24 h. If a positive Coombs test indicates hemolysis, close observation and early treatment with phototherapy or exchange transfusion are needed. Exchange transfusions should be done with type O blood and compatible Rh, and low titer of A and B antigens (Gardner et al. 2020; Verklan et al. 2020).

Hyperbilirubinemia

Bilirubin, the natural byproduct of dying red blood cells, is transported to the liver by binding with albumin. Bound bilirubin is considered non-toxic. The liver conjugates bilirubin to break it down and eliminate it through the stool. If albumin binding sites are saturated, unconjugated bilirubin becomes free bilirubin, circulating in the blood, which can cross the blood–brain barrier and become toxic. As the bilirubin production exceeds the liver's capacity to clear it, jaundice develops. Hyperbilirubinemia is seen with prematurity, small for gestational age (SGA), microcephaly, extravascular blood (such as hematoma and bruising), pallor, petechiae, hepatosplenomegaly, chorioretinitis, and hypothyroidism (Gardner et al. 2020; Verklan et al. 2020).

Hyperbilirubinemia presents several signs, and the most commonly seen is jaundice, which progresses in a cephalocaudal direction. Kernicterus, or bilirubin encephalopathy, is a syndrome of severe brain damage caused by unconjugated bilirubin deposited in the brain cells. Unconjugated bilirubin is highly toxic to neurons because of its fat-soluble affinity for fatty tissues. There is no treatment for kernicterus. Signs of kernicterus are lethargy, hypertonia or hypotonia, poor suck and ability to feed, high-pitched cry, irritability, moderate stupor, hypertonia, inability to handle stimulation, arching of neck or back, fever, deep stupor to coma, and dystonia (Gardner et al. 2020; Verklan et al. 2020).

There are several tests to evaluate hyperbilirubinemia, including total serum bilirubin and direct (conjugated bilirubin). Transcutaneous bilirubin checks are reliable for estimates of serum bilirubin but may limit accuracy depending on skin pigmentation, postnatal age, gestational age, and weight of infant. Blood type and direct Coomb's test are testing for isoimmune hemolytic disease and ABO incompatibility. Other tests done to evaluate hyperbilirubinemia are blood type, hematocrit, Rh, and antibody screen (Gardner et al. 2020; Verklan et al. 2020).

Management of hyperbilirubinemia is essential for the prevention of bilirubin encephalopathy and is dependent on etiology, age, and bilirubin levels. Strategies may include early initiation of feeding, frequent breastfeeding, adequate fluid balance, phototherapy, and exchange transfusion if indicated.

Phototherapy is the use of fluorescent lights on exposed skin, which promotes bilirubin excretion by photoisomerization and alters the structure of bilirubin to a water-soluble form for easier excretion. For effective phototherapy, the neonate's skin must be as exposed as possible to light source, using eye shields to protect the eyes from light. During phototherapy, eye checks should be done with feedings to assess for discharge, pressure, and irritation. There are several potential side effects from phototherapy, such as loose stools, transient skin rashes, hyperthermia, higher metabolic rate, insensible water loss, dehydration, electrolyte imbalances, lethargy, and eye damage (Gardner et al. 2020; Verklan et al. 2020).

Exchange transfusions may be indicated for significant hemolytic disease based on the condition and age of the neonate or if phototherapy fails. An exchange transfusion is done in small aliquots over several hours, removing partially hemolyzed red blood cells and replacing them with donor red blood cells. As the bilirubin is removed, the unbound bilirubin quickly attaches to the unbound donor albumin. Exchange transfusions may cause complications, such as electrolyte and acid–base imbalances, temperature imbalance, necrotizing enterocolitis, vasospasms, thrombi or emboli, infarctions, arrhythmias, volume overload, blood pressure variances, infection, and graft-versus-host disease (Gardner et al. 2020; Verklan et al. 2020).

Congenital Conditions

Congenital conditions, or birth or genetic defects, may require specialized neonatal care. Defects can involve any body system, and are the result of inheritance patterns, chromosomal abnormalities, and multifactorial diseases or disorders. Assessment of the neonate can help identify and diagnose congenital defects, so a complete assessment is needed as soon as possible after birth. A more in-depth examination, such as an ophthalmologic or cardiac consultation, may be needed. Not all genetic defects have signs or features in the neonatal period. Common congenital conditions include Tay-Sachs Disease, trisomies (such as Trisomy 21 or 13), fragile X syndrome, and Turner syndrome. Diagnosis, testing, and management of congenital conditions are variable, based on the specific disorder (Rogelet and Brorsen 2016; Verklan et al. 2020).

Neurological and Neuromuscular Conditions

The neonate is at risk for several types of cranial hemorrhages including extracranial, intraventricular, subdural, subarachnoid, and intracerebellar. Extracranial hemorrhages most commonly include caput succedaneum and cephalohematoma, with subgaleal hemorrhage not as common (see Fig. 1.2). The extracranial hemorrhages are generally related to trauma that occurs during labor and delivery. Caput succedaneum is a serosanguinous, subcutaneous, or extra-periosteal fluid collection with poorly defined margins. Caput can extend across the midline and over suture lines and is associated with head molding. Cephalohematoma is a subperiosteal collection of blood secondary to rupture of the blood vessels between the skull and periosteum. Cephalohematoma is usually well demarcated by suture lines (Rogelet and Brorsen 2016; Verklan et al. 2020).

Intraventricular hemorrhage (IVH) is the most common type of neonatal intracranial hemorrhage and occurs most commonly in the first 72 h of life. There is an increased risk for IVH with lower gestational ages (24–32 weeks) from the presence of the germinal matrix. Other risk factors include fluctuations in blood flow, hyperperfusion, cerebral autoregulation, venous hemodynamics, deficient vascular support, and increased fibrinolytic activity. IVH is graded to four degrees from minimal to most extensive, Grade I-IV IVH. Grades I-II IVH often have no further complications, and are most common. Grades III-IV IVH are the most serious and may result in conditions associated with long-term brain injury to the neonate, such as hydrocephalus and periventricular leukomalacia. Signs of IVH can include decreased motor activity, hypotonia, flaccidity, seizures, apnea and bradycardia, hypotension, bulging fontanel, low hematocrit, and metabolic acidosis. Management of IVH depends on the grade of the hemorrhage, and is mainly supportive to prevent and reduce intracranial pressure. Management includes monitoring, maintaining blood pressure, and preventing coagulopathy (Rogelet and Brorsen 2016; Verklan et al. 2020).

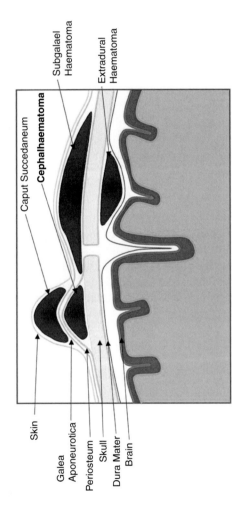

Fig. 1.2 Sites of neonatal extracranial hemorrhages. "Mirza et al. Infected cephalhaematoma causing osteomyelitis: case report and literature review, *Journal of Surgical Case Reports*, Volume 2022, Issue 5, May 2022, rjac225, https://doi.org/10.1093/jscr/rjac225"

Subdural hemorrhage is associated with cerebral contusion from birth trauma, including use of forceps. It is more common in term neonates, and subdural hemorrhage may also be seen with a subarachnoid hemorrhage. Signs of subdural hemorrhage include irritability, focal seizures, stupor, and coma. Management is generally supportive, unless a surgical clot aspiration is required (Rogelet and Brorsen 2016; Verklan et al. 2020).

Subarachnoid hemorrhage is associated with venous blood, trauma, and asphyxia. This type of hemorrhage is more commonly seen in term neonates and is not usually significant. Neonates may be asymptomatic or have an isolated seizure, although a massive hemorrhage will have a rapid and fatal course (Rogelet and Brorsen 2016; Verklan et al. 2020).

An intracerebellar hemorrhage is associated with hypoxia and trauma in VLBW neonates. Signs include apnea, bradycardia, eye deviations, seizures, hydrocephalus, and decreasing hematocrit. This can result in death within 36 h (Rogelet and Brorsen 2016; Verklan et al. 2020).

Hydrocephalus is related to ventricular enlargement where there is an imbalance between formation and absorption of cerebral spinal fluid (CSF). Hydrocephalus is also associated with congenital and acquired lesions. Hydrocephalus is caused by impaired CSF absorption or an overproduction of CSF. Signs of hydrocephalus are increased head circumference, enlarged or bulging fontanels, irritability, poor feeding, little weight gain, vomiting, increased or decreased muscle tone, hyper-reflexes, downward fixation of eyes, and high-pitched cry. Management of hydrocephalus is based on the cause and may include diuretics, CSF removal through lumbar punctures or ventricular taps, surgical removal of obstruction, and surgical placement of a shunt (Rogelet and Brorsen 2016; Verklan et al. 2020).

Hypoxic ischemic encephalopathy (HIE) occurs with a brain injury from a combination of systemic hypoxemia and decreased cerebral perfusion, which leads to ischemia. It is a progressive condition in which asphyxia causes hypoxia, ischemia, and hypercarbia, which in turn leads to cerebral edema and circulatory disturbances. Persistent asphyxia leads to tissue necrosis and cerebral edema. HIE is associated with various conditions, but most commonly IVH. Other conditions include abruptio placenta, placenta previa, post-maturity, prolapsed or nuchal cord, intrauterine growth retardation (IUGR), maternal blood pressure abnormalities or cardiopulmonary disease, abnormal uterine contractions, and maternal hypoxia. Signs of HIE are associated with the degree of the condition and may include lethargy, jitteriness, hypersensitivity, apnea, decreased tone, decreased spontaneous movement, seizures, stupor, coma, severe hypertonia, constant and exaggerated movements, altered eye movements, and a poor or absent Moro reflex. Management of HIE is mainly supportive and includes maintaining oxygenation and ventilation, treating and preventing seizures, treating any electrolyte imbalances, fluid management, and minimizing hypotension, hypoxia, acidosis, and severe apnea and bradycardia. Therapeutic hypothermia may also be a strategy for those neonates who meet criteria (Rogelet and Brorsen 2016; Verklan et al. 2020).

Periventricular leukomalacia (PVL) is an ischemic brain lesion that is usually bilateral, and may be present at birth from antepartum injury. PVL is most commonly seen in premature neonates associated with an IVH. PVL is a manifestation of HIE from reduced oxygen delivery to vulnerable areas of the brain. Signs of PVL cystic lesions are spastic diplegia, leg diplegia, visual deficits, and hydrocephalus may be present. There is no current management of PVL, but the sequelae can be managed (Rogelet and Brorsen 2016; Verklan et al. 2020).

Cardiac Disorders

Congenital heart disease (CHD) involves anatomic malformation(s) that develop in utero. There is a high risk for CHD with maternal diabetes, teratogen exposure, advanced maternal age, small for gestational age, very low and extremely low birthweights, prematurity, and chromosome anomalies. Signs of CHD do not always occur immediately after birth and are usually seen within the first 2 weeks of life. Cyanotic heart defects may not show signs until the ductus arteriosus closes. Cyanotic heart defects have decreased pulmonary blood flow, a right to left shunt, a right outflow obstruction from the heart is present, and there is cyanosis. General signs of cyanotic heart defects include right-sided heart failure, hepatomegaly, metabolic acidosis, poor perfusion, hypoglycemia, a murmur may be present, prominent right ventricle and atria, and oligemic lung fields. Acyanotic heart defects may have signs including pulmonary symptoms of congestive heart failure, murmur, metabolic acidosis, hypoglycemia, cardiomegaly, and pulmonary edema. CHD may not be immediately diagnosed, although defects may be detected in utero with ultrasound. Testing may include electrocardiogram (ECG), hyperoxia test, and echocardiogram (Gardner et al. 2020; Rogelet and Brorsen 2016).

Transposition of the great arteries (TGA), also known as transposition of the great vessels, is a cyanotic defect in which there is an inversion of parallel tubes in embryonic development, and the transposed arteries create two parallel circulations. In TGA the aorta carries desaturated blood back to the systemic circulation and the pulmonary artery carries oxygenated blood back to the lungs (see Fig. 1.3). Survival occurs with a patent ductus arteriosus in addition to communication at the atrial/ventricular level to allow oxygenated blood to reach the body. Management of TGA may include the use of prostaglandin immunoglobulin to maintain a PDA, maintain and correct electrolytes, a balloon atrioseptostomy, and an arterial switch as the final repair (Gardner et al. 2020; Rogelet and Brorsen 2016).

Tricuspid atresia is another cyanotic heart defect which occurs when there is no development of the valve between right atrium and ventricle (see Fig. 1.4). Signs of tricuspid atresia depend on the presence and size of septal communication. A murmur may or may not be present. Management of tricuspid atresia may include a surgical Blalock-Taussig (BT) shunt implant between the subclavian and pulmonary arteries, pulmonary artery banding, and a Fontan procedure, which is the corrective repair (Gardner et al. 2020; Rogelet and Brorsen 2016).

An additional cyanotic heart defect is tetralogy of Fallot, which actually has multiple defects (see Fig. 1.5). These defects are pulmonary atresia or stenosis, right ventricular hypertrophy, an overriding aorta, and a large ventricular septal defect (VSD). Tetralogy of Fallot may not be seen in the neonatal period if there is ade-

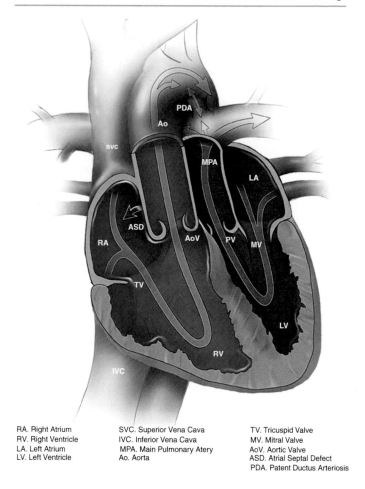

RA. Right Atrium
RV. Right Ventricle
LA. Left Atrium
LV. Left Ventricle

SVC. Superior Vena Cava
IVC. Inferior Vena Cava
MPA. Main Pulmonary Atery
Ao. Aorta

TV. Tricuspid Valve
MV. Mitral Valve
AoV. Aortic Valve
ASD. Atrial Septal Defect
PDA. Patent Ductus Arteriosis

Fig. 1.3 Transposition of the great arteries. Centers for disease control and prevention, national center on birth defects and developmental disabilities. https://www.cdc.gov/ncbddd/heartdefects/d-tga.html

Tricuspid Atresia

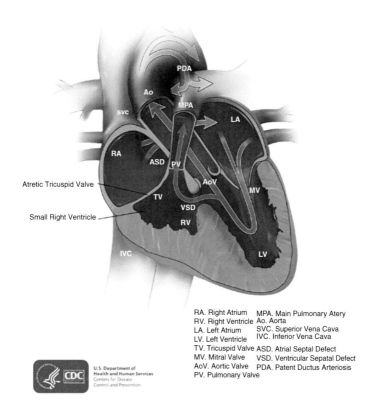

RA. Right Atrium   MPA. Main Pulmonary Atery
RV. Right Ventricle Ao. Aorta
LA. Left Atrium   SVC. Superior Vena Cava
LV. Left Ventricle IVC. Inferior Vena Cava
TV. Tricuspid Valve ASD. Atrial Septal Defect
MV. Mitral Valve   VSD. Ventricular Sepatal Defect
AoV. Aortic Valve PDA. Patent Ductus Arteriosis
PV. Pulmonary Valve

Fig. 1.4 Tricuspid atresia. Centers for disease control and prevention, national center on birth defects and developmental disabilities. https://www.cdc.gov/ncbddd/heartdefects/tricuspid-atresia.html

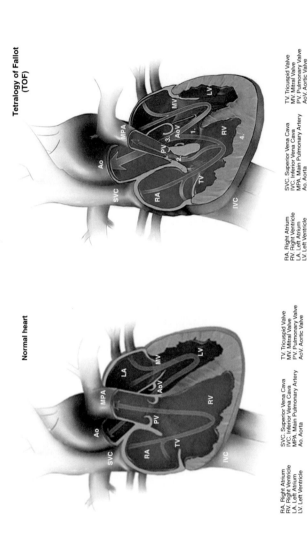

Fig. 1.5 Tetralogy of Fallot. Centers for disease control and prevention, national center on birth defects and developmental disabilities. https://www.cdc.gov/ncbddd/heartdefects/tetralogyoffallot.html

quate mixing of oxygenated and unoxygenated blood and shunts for blood flow. Management of tetralogy of Fallot includes metabolic and volume management, use of PGE to maintain the patency of a PDA, a BT shunt, between subclavian and pulmonary arteries, and closure of the VSD with a patch (Gardner et al. 2020; Rogelet and Brorsen 2016).

Another cyanotic heart defect is truncus arteriosus, where one artery forms both the pulmonary artery and the aorta in utero (see Fig. 1.6). With this condition, mixed blood is pumped to the body. A VSD is almost always associated with truncus arteriosus. Management of truncus arteriosus includes treatment of congestive heart failure, creating a graft between the right ventricle and pulmonary artery, pulmonary artery banding, and closure of the VSD (Gardner et al. 2020; Rogelet and Brorsen 2016).

Total anomalous pulmonary venous return (TAPVR) is another cyanotic heart defect where when the pulmonary veins drain into the right atrium instead of the left atrium (see Fig. 1.7). Management of TAPVR is to create communication between the right and left sides of the heart to survive, closure of a PDA, and detachment of anomalous veins with transplantation to the left atrium (Gardner et al. 2020; Rogelet and Brorsen 2016).

Pulmonary stenosis and pulmonary atresia are also cyanotic heart defects. Pulmonary stenosis refers to the narrowing of the pulmonary valve, while pulmonary atresia is a malformation of the valve. These conditions increase the pressure in the right side of the heart, causing right ventricular hypertrophy, and may have a VSD as well. Management of pulmonary atresia or stenosis includes correcting metabolic imbalances, maintaining a PDA by using PGE, an atrial septectomy, pulmonary valvotomy, right ventricular outflow tract reconstruction and patching, and a Fontan procedure (Gardner et al. 2020; Rogelet and Brorsen 2016).

Patent ductus arteriosus (PDA) is when the ductus fails to close, which is influenced by hypoxia and acidosis. The amount and direction of blood shunting through a PDA depends on

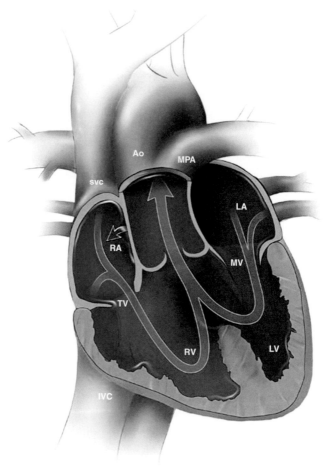

RA. Right Atrium	SVC. Superior Vena Cava	TV. Tricuspid Valve
RV. Right Ventricle	IVC. Inferior Vena Cava	MV. Mitral Valve
LA. Left Atrium	MPA. Main Pulmonary Atery	
LV. Left Ventricle	Ao. Aorta	

Fig. 1.6 Truncus arteriosus. Centers for disease control and prevention, national center on birth defects and developmental disabilities. https://www. cdc.gov/ncbddd/heartdefects/truncusarteriosus.html

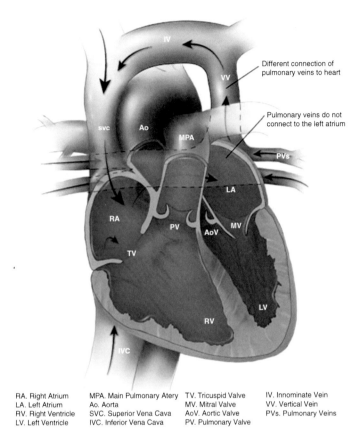

RA. Right Atrium	MPA. Main Pulmonary Atery	TV. Tricuspid Valve	IV. Innominate Vein
LA. Left Atrium	Ao. Aorta	MV. Mitral Valve	VV. Vertical Vein
RV. Right Ventricle	SVC. Superior Vena Cava	AoV. Aortic Valve	PVs. Pulmonary Veins
LV. Left Ventricle	IVC. Inferior Vena Cava	PV. Pulmonary Valve	

Fig. 1.7 Total anomalous pulmonary venous return. Centers for disease control and prevention, national center on birth defects and developmental disabilities. https://www.cdc.gov/ncbddd/heartdefects/tapvr.html

peripheral and systemic vascular resistance and the size of the PDA. Signs include murmur, widened pulse pressure, bounding or full pulses, fluctuations in oxygen requirements, and pulmonary congestion and edema. Management of patent ductus arteriosus includes fluid and nutrition management, medications to close the ductus (indomethacin, ibuprofen, or acetaminophen), surgical ligation, and ventilation and cardiotropic support in severe cases (Gardner et al. 2020; Rogelet and Brorsen 2016).

Persistent pulmonary hypertension (PPHN) happens when there isn't a normal increase in systemic vascular resistance (SVR) and a decrease in pulmonary vascular resistance (PVR) after birth. Asphyxia, hypoxia, acidosis, and other complications cause an increase in PVR. PPHN is also associated with hypoglycemia, hypocalcemia, hyperviscosity syndrome, sepsis, term or post-term gestation. Risk factors for PPHN are intrauterine closure of the ductus, abnormal responsiveness of the pulmonary vasculature to hypoxia, repeated intrauterine hypoxia, regional alveolar hypoxia, congenital diaphragmatic hernia, pulmonary hypoplasia, alterations in vasoactive mediator levels, microthrombus formation in the pulmonary vascular bed, and meconium aspiration syndrome (MAS). A PDA with a right-to-left shunt also occurs with PPHN. Signs of PPHN may include murmur, oligemic lung fields, respiratory distress, hypotension, hypoxia, hypercarbia, acidosis, hypoglycemia, cyanosis, metabolic acidosis, and a difference between preductal and post-ductal PaO_2. There are specific considerations for treating PPHN. Management of PPHN may include neutral thermal environment, low stiumulation and minimal handling, maintaining hemoglobin and fluid and electrolytes, vasopressors, sedation, paralytics, high-frequency ventilation (HFV), nitric oxide (NO), and extracorporeal membrane oxygenation (ECMO) (Gardner et al. 2020; Rogelet and Brorsen 2016).

An atrial septal defect (ASD) occurs when there is a defect between the atria (see Fig. 1.8). Oxygenated blood shunts through ASD from left to right, and mixes with deoxygenated blood. ASD has minor effects on circulatory status and is usually found with other heart defects. Neonates with ASD may be asymptomatic, have a murmur, dyspnea, or fatigue. ASDs generally close on their own, although a patch can be used or, rarely, surgical closure (Gardner et al. 2020; Rogelet and Brorsen 2016).

A ventricular septal defect (VSD) is when there is a defect between the ventricles with mixing of blood (see Fig. 1.9). This

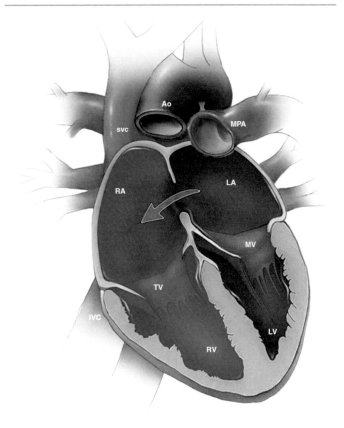

RA. Right Atrium   SVC. Superior Vena Cava   TV. Tricuspid Valve
RV. Right Ventricle   IVC. Inferior Vena Cava   MV. Mitral Valve
LA. Left Atrium   MPA. Main Pulmonary Atery
LV. Left Ventricle   Ao. Aorta

Fig. 1.8 Atrial septal defect. Centers for disease control and prevention, national center on birth defects and developmental disabilities. https://www.cdc.gov/ncbddd/heartdefects/atrialseptaldefect.html

may minimally impact circulation unless the VSD is large enough to cause congestive heart failure (CHF) from pulmonary over-circulation. Neonates with a VSD may be asymptomatic, or may

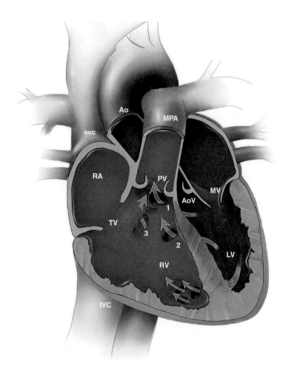

RA. Right Atrium	SVC. Superior Vena Cava	TV. Tricuspid Valve	1. Conoventricular, malaligned
RV. Right Ventricle	IVC. Inferior Vena Cava	MV. Mitral Valve	2. perimemnranous
LA. Left Atrium	MPA. Main Pulmonary Atery	PV. Pulmonary Valve	3. inlet
LV. Left Ventricle	Ao. Aorta	AoV. Aortic Valve	4. muscular

Fig. 1.9 Ventricular septal defect. Centers for disease control and prevention, national center on birth defects and developmental disabilities. https://www.cdc.gov/ncbddd/heartdefects/ventricularseptaldefect.html

have a murmur, poor weight gain, and fatigue. The defect may close on its own without treatment. CHF may necessitate VSD repair through a patch or surgical closure (Gardner et al. 2020; Rogelet and Brorsen 2016).

Coarctation of the aorta occurs is the constriction or narrowing of the aorta and may be pre- or post-ductal (see Fig. 1.10). A PDA is needed to maintain the systemic circulation as a result of diminished perfusion to body after the narrowing in the aorta. There is a difference in upper and lower limb perfusion, (the main sign of coarctation), which may not be present until after the ductus has closed. Signs of coarctation of the aorta include pallor, dyspnea, irritability, and sweating. Management is correcting the narrowing of the aorta through balloon angiography, stent placement, surgical reconstruction, or patching (Gardner et al. 2020; Rogelet and Brorsen 2016).

Hypoplastic left heart syndrome (HLHS) is primarily the underdevelopment of the left ventricle, but may also include other left-sided underdevelopment such as stenosis of the mitral and aortic valves and hypoplasia of the aorta (see Fig. 1.11). A small left ventricle causes inability to maintain adequate cardiac output and the PDA is the main source of systemic blood flow. There may not be symptoms initially if there is a PDA and a patent foramen ovale. However signs may develop including pallor, cyanosis, dyspnea, weak pulse, and hypotension. HLHS is managed depending on the severity and associated morbidities. Management includes a heart transplant or a three-stage surgery. In some cases palliative care may be the only option (Gardner et al. 2020; Rogelet and Brorsen 2016).

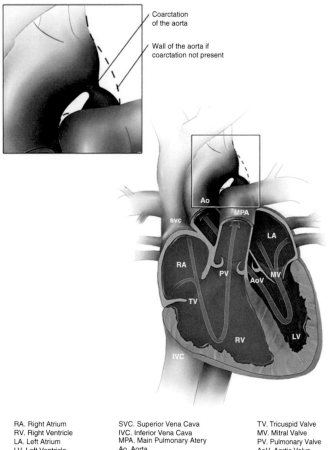

RA. Right Atrium
RV. Right Ventricle
LA. Left Atrium
LV. Left Ventricle

SVC. Superior Vena Cava
IVC. Inferior Vena Cava
MPA. Main Pulmonary Atery
Ao. Aorta

TV. Tricuspid Valve
MV. Mitral Valve
PV. Pulmonary Valve
AoV. Aortic Valve

Fig. 1.10 Coarctation of the aorta. Centers for disease control and prevention, national center on birth defects and developmental disabilities. https://www.cdc.gov/ncbddd/heartdefects/coarctationofaorta.html

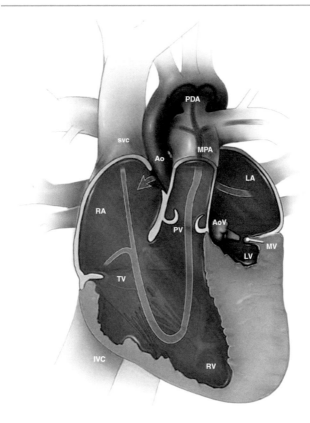

RA. Right Atrium	SVC. Superior Vena Cava	TV. Tricuspid Valve
RV. Right Ventricle	IVC. Inferior Vena Cava	MV. Mitral Valve
LA. Left Atrium	MPA. Main Pulmonary Atery	PV. Pulmonary Valve
LV. Left Ventricle	Ao. Aorta	AoV. Aortic Valve
	PDA. Patent Ductus Arteriosis	

Fig. 1.11 Hypoplastic left heart syndrome. Centers for disease control and prevention, national center on birth defects and developmental disabilities. https://www.cdc.gov/ncbddd/heartdefects/hlhs.html

Blood Gas Abnormalities

Respiratory acidosis is an imbalance that is caused by an impaired pulmonary process which interferes with gas exchange. Causes of respiratory acidosis include asphyxia, hypoventilation, respiratory distress syndrome (RDS), transient tachypnea of the newborn (TTNB), meconium aspiration (MAS), pneumonia, pneumothorax, congenital heart defects, congestive heart failure, central depression due to intraventricular hemorrhage (IVH), medications, and neurological disorders. Blood gas values include decreased pH, increased pCO_2, and normal HCO_3, and BE. Signs of respiratory acidosis are apnea, respiratory distress, irritability, and lethargy. Management of respiratory acidosis may include increased ventilation to blow off excess carbon dioxide (Gardner et al. 2020; Verklan et al. 2020).

Respiratory alkalosis is an imbalance driven by the respiratory system caused by hyperventilation, tachypnea, fever, abnormal neurological response, response to hypoxia, or maternal heroin addiction. Blood gas values include increased pH, decreased pCO_2, and a normal HCO_3 and BE. Respiratory alkalosis signs include lethargy, decreased muscle tone, and tachypnea. Management is correcting the causative condition (Gardner et al. 2020; Verklan et al. 2020).

Metabolic acidosis is an imbalance driven by the metabolic system caused by depleted sodium bicarbonate, excessive acid production, decreased acid excretion, hypoxia from lactic acidosis, inborn errors of metabolism, TPN administration, diarrhea, renal tubular acidosis, and acetazolamide. Blood gas values include decreased pH, normal pCO_2, and decreased HCO_3 and BE. Signs of metabolic acidosis may include lethargy, irritability, and tachypnea. Management is focused on correcting the cause and sodium bicarbonate may be given in some circumstances (Gardner et al. 2020; Verklan et al. 2020).

Metabolic alkalosis is an imbalance caused by a loss of hydrogen chloride or potassium, excessive alkali intake, bicarb or acetate administration, gastric suctioning, and diuretics. Blood gas values include increased pH, normal pCO_2, and increased HCO_3

and BE. Signs are muscle spasms, jitteriness, and lethargy. Management is correcting the causative condition (Gardner et al. 2020; Verklan et al. 2020).

Respiratory Conditions

There are many neonatal conditions that can impact oxygenation and ventilation. Physical defects can affect airways. Choanal atresia is a condition where the tissue narrows or blocks the nasal airway. Choanal atresia is the most common nasal abnormality in newborn infants. However, the cause remains unclear. Choanal atresia causes difficulty breathing, and the neonate may need an alternate airway or intubation (Gardner et al. 2020; Verklan et al. 2020).

Another physical defect is micrognathia, which is a small jaw with a tongue which tends to ball up at the back of the mouth and fall back toward the throat. This defect causes difficulty breathing and is related to syndromes and other conditions (Gardner et al. 2020; Verklan et al. 2020).

Cleft lip and palate occur when a baby's lip or mouth does not form properly during pregnancy, and may occur separately or combined. Clefts can interfere with the ability of the neonate to breathe, cause feeding problems, and make them susceptible to ear infections. Surgical repair is required, which may require several surgeries (Gardner et al. 2020; Verklan et al. 2020).

Tracheoesophageal fistula (TEF) occurs when an abnormal channel connects the trachea to the esophagus. Liquid can get into the trachea and lungs through this fistula, which can cause coughing and choking. This defect may cause lung infections such as pneumonia and requires surgical repair. TEF may be associated with esophageal atresia (Gardner et al. 2020; Verklan et al. 2020).

Esophageal atresia (EA) occurs when the esophagus does not form completely. Severe atresia can cause a closure of the esophagus, which results in the inability for any oral intake to make it to the stomach. EA may occur with or without TEF, and this defect requires surgical repair (Gardner et al. 2020; Verklan et al. 2020).

Tracheal stenosis or atresia occurs when there is narrowing or constriction of the trachea, and may be congenital or acquired by trauma. This defect restricts the neonate's ability to breathe normally. Signs include wheezing, coughing, dyspnea, apnea, cyanosis, or acrocyanosis. Surgical repair is needed (Gardner et al. 2020; Verklan et al. 2020).

Congenital diaphragmatic hernia (CDH) is a defect in the diaphragm in which the abdominal organs can move into the chest cavity and compress the lung. With CDH a bag and mask should not be used for resuscitation and the neonate must be intubated as soon as possible. Management also includes insertion of an oral or nasal gastric tube to decompress the gastrointestinal tract. CDH requires surgical repair (Gardner et al. 2020; Verklan et al. 2020).

Tracheomalacia is an abnormal collapse of the tracheal walls that may be congenital. This, can be isolated or found in combination with other lesions that cause compression or damage to the airway. The tracheal walls are soft and collapse during respiration. The condition is usually benign, with symptoms due to airway obstruction, and improves as the neonate grows. Signs of tracheomalacia can include dyspnea, upper respiratory infections, stridor, and rales. Management is the use of humidified air, careful feedings, and antibiotics for infections (Gardner et al. 2020; Verklan et al. 2020).

Apnea is the cessation of breathing for greater than 20 seconds, or less if accompanied by bradycardia. Risk factors include prematurity, VLBW, ELBW, birth asphyxia, IVH, maternal sedation, seizures, central nervous system depression, and respiratory distress. Apnea may be central, obstructive, or mixed. Central apnea is related to the immaturity of the central respiratory drive, which causes a lack of breathing coordination. Obstructive apnea is when an airway or nasal obstruction does not allow airflow. Mixed apnea is a combination of both central and obstructive apnea at the same time. Apnea is also associated with underlying conditions, such as pulmonary air leaks, sepsis, anemia, gastro-esophageal reflux disease (GERD), necrotizing enterocolitis (NEC), patent ductus arteriosus (PDA), hemorrhagic shock, metabolic abnormalities, hyperthermia, and hypothermia. Management of apnea may include treatment of the causative condition, maintain oxygen saturation, minimize vagal stimulation, maintain a neutral temperature environment, blood transfusions, continuous positive airway pressure (CPAP), medications such as caffeine and aminophylline, and mechanical ventilation (Gardner et al. 2020; Verklan et al. 2020).

Transient tachypnea of the newborn (TTNB or TTN) occurs when there is delayed absorption of fetal lung fluid following delivery. Risk factors are prematurity, SGA, C-section, and precipitous delivery. Signs of TTNB are tachypnea, retractions, grunting, nasal flaring, color changes, and crackles on auscultation. TTNB usually resolves within the first 72 h of life, and supportive management includes oxygen, fluids, minimal handling, and neutral thermal environment. In rare cases, CPAP or mechanical ventilation is required (Gardner et al. 2020; Verklan et al. 2020).

Respiratory distress syndrome (RDS) occurs with alveolar collapse caused by insufficient surfactant production, primarily with prematurity. Surfactant lowers the surface tension of the alveolar membrane and without surfactant, the alveoli collapse at the end of each expiration. Signs of RDS are tachypnea, retractions, grunting, shallow respirations, nasal flaring, apnea, color changes, and edema. Management of RDS is initial resuscitation, oxygen, surfactant, and possibly mechanical ventilation (Gardner et al. 2020; Verklan et al. 2020).

A pulmonary air leak occurs when air escapes out of the normal pulmonary air space. Causes of air leaks may be increased inspiratory pressures with mechanical ventilation due to poor lung compliance, or air trapping from meconium aspiration. Risk factors for air leaks include respiratory distress syndrome, mechanical ventilation, pneumonia and related sepsis, meconium aspiration, amniotic fluid aspiration, congenital deformities, and direct trauma to airway (Gardner et al. 2020; Verklan et al. 2020).

A pneumothorax occurs when air escapes into the pleural space, and is commonly caused by increased inspiratory pressures and inconsistent ventilation of the lungs. A pneumothorax can cause apnea, bradycardia, hypotension, and cardiovascular collapse. Signs may be increasing tachypnea, grunting and nasal flaring, retractions, cyanosis, displaced point of maximum intensity (PMI), asymmetrical chest expansion, diminished or distant breath sounds on the affected side, and unexplained changes in oxygenation and ventilation. Management of pneumothorax may include close observation, increased oxygen concentration, needle aspiration, or chest tube insertion (Gardner et al. 2020; Verklan et al. 2020).

Pulmonary interstitial emphysema (PIE) occurs when air escapes from the ruptured alveolar ducts into external pleural layers, subpleural space, lymphatic, and venous circulation. Risk factors include respiratory distress and mechanical ventilation, especially with high peak pressures. PIE can cause pneumothorax, pneumopericardium, and air embolus. Signs of PIE may be tachypnea, dyspnea, hypotension, bradycardia, hypercarbia, hypoxia, and acidosis. Management of PIE may include supportive measures, use of high-frequency ventilation, positioning of the neonate, selective intubation, and ventilation. Surgical resection may be needed if PIE is not resolved (Gardner et al. 2020; Verklan et al. 2020).

Chronic lung disease (CLD) occurs with oxygen and positive-pressure ventilation use in neonates who are premature and VLBW or ELBW. Prolonged mechanical ventilation or use of high pressures cause volutrauma and barotrauma. CLD can create pulmonary hypertension, abnormal pulmonary vascular development, inflammation and scarring of injured lung tissue, increased airway resistance, decreased lung compliance, increased airway reactivity, and increased airway obstruction. The main goal is prevention of CLD. Strategies include weaning off ventilation, using minimal pressures, surfactant, bronchodilators, steroids, diuretics, restricted fluids, and supportive nutrition (Gardner et al. 2020; Verklan et al. 2020).

Meconium aspiration syndrome (MAS) is common with fetal distress. The fetus passes meconium prior to delivery and aspirates this into the lungs. Signs are respiratory distress and cyanosis. MAS can result in air leaks, PPHN, and airway obstruction. Management of MAS includes initial resuscitation, oxygenation, surfactant, antibiotics, correction of metabolic disturbances, cautious handling, neutral thermal environment, sedation, ventilation with the lowest possible pressures, and high-frequency ventilation (Gardner et al. 2020; Verklan et al. 2020).

Gastrointestinal and Genitourinary Disorders

Duodenal atresia is a congenital condition in which a portion of the duodenum lumen is absent or closed. It is associated with Trisomy 21. Signs of duodenal atresia are bile-stained vomiting, upper abdomen distention, and large amounts of gastric aspirate prior to feeding. This defect requires surgical repair (Rogelet and Brorsen 2016; Verklan et al. 2020).

Pyloric stenosis is a narrowing of the pyloric orifice, usually with a palpable pyloric mass. Signs include feeding intolerance, vomiting, and upper abdomen distention. Stenosis usually presents at 2–3 weeks of life with vomiting and requires surgical intervention (Rogelet and Brorsen 2016; Verklan et al. 2020).

Meconium ileus is associated with cystic fibrosis, and occurs when no meconium is passed through the rectum. Signs are feeding intolerance, vomiting, general abdominal distention, and an inability to pass meconium. Management can include use of contrast enemas or surgery if the obstruction is not relieved (Rogelet and Brorsen 2016; Verklan et al. 2020).

Imperforate anus is a malformation of the anorectal tract without a rectal opening. The rectum can end in a blind pouch or have openings to the bladder, urethra, vaginal, or scrotal areas, or have a fistula on the perineum. Management requires dilation of the perineal fistula if present, surgical repair, and a temporary colostomy (Rogelet and Brorsen 2016; Verklan et al. 2020).

Volvulus is a twisting of the intestines that occurs during fetal development, which results in obstruction and impeded blood flow to those organs. Signs are clear vomiting that changes to bile, bloody stools, abdominal distention, shock, and sepsis. Management is surgical intervention, and obstruction is a medical emergency (Rogelet and Brorsen 2016; Verklan et al. 2020).

Meconium or mucus plug syndrome occurs when the intestine becomes obstructed from meconium, mucus plug, or both. Risk factors are prematurity, maternal diabetes, and neonates with small left colon which becomes obstructed with meconium. Management includes the use of glycerin suppositories, diluted normal saline enema, and gentle rectal stimulus (Rogelet and Brorsen 2016; Verklan et al. 2020).

Hirschsprung's disease causes a blockage of the large intestine due to improper peristalsis. Signs are inability to pass meconium, abdominal distention, malabsorption, and chronic constipation. Management includes surgical resection, removal of the abnormal colon, and a colostomy may be needed (Rogelet and Brorsen 2016; Verklan et al. 2020).

Necrotizing enterocolitis (NEC) is an acquired disease of intestinal necrosis, which may be caused by decreased blood flow to the bowel that prevents the bowel from producing the normal protective mucus. Risk factors for developing NEC, are prematurity, VLBW and ELBW, immaturity of the gastrointestinal tract, compromised intrauterine placental blood flow, congenital heart disease, PDA, maternal cocaine abuse, and use of concentrated formulas. Signs of NEC may include respiratory distress, apnea, lethargy, irritability, decreased peripheral perfusion, inability to regulate temperature, feeding intolerance, increased abdominal circumference, visible intestinal loops, abdominal discoloration, distention, tenderness, occult or frank blood in stools, vomiting of blood, decreased or absent bowel sounds, localized abdominal mass, ascites, cardiovascular collapse, and shock. Severe NEC can lead to neonatal death. There are medical and surgical management strategies for NEC. Medical management includes respiratory support, IV fluids, discontinuing feedings, vasopressors, sodium bicarbonate for acidosis, insertion of nasogastric (NG) tube to low intermittent suction for gastric decompression, TPN, transfusions of blood or blood products, strict intake and output, and diligent assessments. Surgical management can include resection of the necrotic bowel with an ileostomy or colostomy which may be temporary (Rogelet and Brorsen 2016; Verklan et al. 2020).

An omphalocele is an abdominal wall defect with protrusion of the abdominal contents into the base of the umbilical cord. Management includes covering and protecting the exposed abdominal contents, NG tube placement, cardiopulmonary support, electrolyte management, and surgical repair (Rogelet and Brorsen 2016; Verklan et al. 2020).

Gastroschisis is a congenital anomaly where the intestines or other organs protrude through a defect in the abdominal wall. Management includes covering and protecting exposed abdominal contents, NG tube, cardiopulmonary support, electrolyte management, and surgical repair (Rogelet and Brorsen 2016; Verklan et al. 2020).

Cloacal exstrophy is a complex anomaly that affects the gastrointestinal and genitourinary systems. The anomaly includes omphaloceles, exstrophy (protrusion) of the bladder through the abdominal wall, imperforate anus, and spinal defects. Management includes covering the exposed contents, providing intravenous fluids, and surgical management (Rogelet and Brorsen 2016; Verklan et al. 2020).

Multicystic dysplastic kidney is a condition caused by the malformation of the kidney during fetal development. Although the affected kidney does not function, most neonates are asymptomatic. Surgical removal of the multicystic dysplastic kidney is done with hypertension, infection, or respiratory compromise (Rogelet and Brorsen 2016; Verklan et al. 2020).

Polycystic kidney disease is an inherited disorder where clusters of cysts develop in the kidneys. Signs may include bilateral, smooth, enlarged kidneys, renal insufficiency, renal failure, and hypertension. Polycystic kidneys are associated with oligohydramnios, pulmonary hypoplasia, and Potter's syndrome. This condition may be fatal, and a kidney transplant may be eventually needed (Rogelet and Brorsen 2016; Verklan et al. 2020).

Acute kidney injury happens from a sudden decline in kidney function, and can cause imbalances in fluid, electrolytes, and waste products. Risk factors for acute kidney injury are some maternal medications, prematurity, VLBW or ELBW, asphyxia, need for resuscitation, low APGAR scores, meningitis, electrolyte imbalance, sepsis, and nephrotoxic medication exposure.

Management includes maintaining fluid and electrolytes, monitoring intake and output, and treatment of underlying conditions (Rogelet and Brorsen 2016; Verklan et al. 2020).

Renal failure occurs when the kidneys lose the ability to remove waste and balance fluids from prerenal, intrinsic, or postrenal disorders. Kidney hypoperfusion causes prerenal failure which can lead to intrinsic renal damage. Obstruction to urinary flow in kidneys causes postrenal failure. Signs of acute renal failure may include oliguria, anuria, hematuria, proteinuria, fluid overload, hypertension, cardiac dysrhythmias, tachypnea, cardiomegaly, heart failure, irritability, lethargy, seizures, and failure to thrive. Management of acute renal failure includes fluid and electrolyte management, vitamin D supplementation, diuretics, dialysis, and blood pressure maintenance (Rogelet and Brorsen 2016; Verklan et al. 2020).

A urinary tract infection (UTI) may cause asymptomatic bacteriuria, pyelonephritis, or sepsis. Signs of a UTI are fever, poor weight gain, poor feeding, unexplained prolonged jaundice, or signs of sepsis. UTI management is the use of anti-infectives (Rogelet and Brorsen 2016; Verklan et al. 2020).

An inguinal hernia is intestines bulging through a weak part in the inguinal canal, and is commonly seen in males and with prolonged mechanical ventilation. Management includes respiratory support as needed, and surgical repair (Rogelet and Brorsen 2016; Verklan et al. 2020).

Testicular torsion is a twisting of the spermatic cord that supplies blood to the testicle. Signs are usually a non-tender, firm, swollen, and cyanotic testicle, which may be necrotic. Surgical repair is needed (Rogelet and Brorsen 2016; Verklan et al. 2020).

Ambiguous genitalia is rare and is where neonatal external genitals are not clearly either male or female. Genitals may not be well-formed, there may be characteristics of both sexes, or external sex organs do not match the internal sex organs or genetic sex. Ambiguous genitalia requires consultations for management and decisions about gender determination (Rogelet and Brorsen 2016; Verklan et al. 2020).

Musculoskeletal Conditions

There are many musculoskeletal conditions that can be seen with neonates. Skull fractures usually occur from birth trauma, and may be linear or depressed. Signs of skull fractures are edema, abrasion, hematoma, palpable bony irregularity, obvious skull deformity, vomiting, irritability, and lethargy. Management includes pain and intracranial pressure management. Management of uncomplicated linear fractures is supportive but may require medical or surgical interventions if associated with a dural tear. Surgical elevation may be required with depressed skull fractures (Gardner et al. 2020; Verklan et al. 2020).

Clavicular fractures can happen as a result of birth trauma, associated with shoulder dystocia, breech deliveries, and macrosomia. Signs of clavicular fractures are crepitus, palpable bony irregularity, muscle spasm, and pseudo-paralysis due to pain from moving. Management includes pain management, support of the affected arm, and limiting movement while healing (Gardner et al. 2020; Verklan et al. 2020).

Birth trauma may also cause facial and mandibular fractures, particularly with forceps and breech deliveries. Signs are edema, abrasion, hematoma, palpable bony irregularity or obvious deformity, vomiting, and irritability. Management includes pain management, support, and surgical intervention (Gardner et al. 2020; Verklan et al. 2020).

Long bone fractures also happen from birth trauma, which may include the humerus or femur. Risk factors are breech presentation, shoulder presentation, and congenital hypotonia. Signs of long bone fracture include loss of spontaneous limb movement, edema, and pain with a passive range of motion. Management includes pain management, splinting, closed reduction, casting, traction, and suspension (Gardner et al. 2020; Verklan et al. 2020).

Torticollis is when the head is in a tilted position and there is limited movement of the neck from involvement of the sternocleidomastoid (SCM) muscle. Torticollis may be caused by an abnormal position in utero, maternal fibrosis, or stretching of the neck during delivery. Management of torticollis includes repositioning the head in the opposite direction, using sandbags or other support for positioning, passive stretching, and rotating the head. Physical therapy or surgical interventions may be warranted later in life (Gardner et al. 2020; Verklan et al. 2020).

Birth trauma can cause brachial plexus injuries from macrosomia, shoulder dystocia, and breech presentation. Signs are abnormal positioning, palsy, abnormal reflexes, and flaccidity of the affected arm. Management of brachial plexus injuries is supportive (Gardner et al. 2020; Verklan et al. 2020).

Polydactyly is the presence of one or more extra digits which can affect hands, feet, or both. Management of polydactyly depends on the extent of the condition. Ligation can be done of a digit without a bone, which causes necrosis and then the digit can be removed. A digit with a bone requires surgical removal (Gardner et al. 2020; Verklan et al. 2020).

Syndactyly is webbing or fusion between digits which can affect hands, feet, or both. This condition can also be due to genetic or unknown causes. Syndactyly may involve tissue only, or could also involve bones and nails, and can also be found in conjunction with other congenital anomalies or syndromes. Management of syndactyly is surgical repair (Gardner et al. 2020; Verklan et al. 2020).

Scoliosis can be congenital or idiopathic and is an abnormal curvature of the spine. Congenital scoliosis is a lateral curve of the spine associated with vertebral anomalies. Signs of scoliosis include subclinical curvatures, neurological complications, pulmonary restriction, cor pulmonale, and premature death. Management of scoliosis may include bracing or surgical repair (Gardner et al. 2020; Verklan et al. 2020).

Developmental hip dysplasia is the abnormal formation of the hip joint that causes an unstable hip, which may be associated with twisting of the femur and contractures. Subluxable hip dysplasia is when the ball of the hip move around loosely in the hip joint, while dislocated hip dysplasia is when the ball of the hip slides in and out of the joint. Hip dysplasia is caused by maternal hormones and abnormal fetal position. Management can be medical or surgical, including exercise, support (such as a harness), and open reduction (Gardner et al. 2020; Verklan et al. 2020).

Metatarsus adductus is the most common foot deformity where the metatarsus bones rest in an adductive position, causing the middle of the foot to bend toward the body. Management includes passive exercise, alignment, and casting (Gardner et al. 2020; Verklan et al. 2020).

Clubfoot or talipes equinovarus is a common congenital anomaly where the foot has a curled shape or is twisted which includes the ankle, heel, and toes. Management may include manipulation, casting, and surgical correction (Gardner et al. 2020; Verklan et al. 2020).

Osteomyelitis and septic arthritis occur when bacteria embed itself into the bone or joint from contaminated skin. Prevention is essential, with good skin care and using aseptic and sterile techniques for procedures. Signs of osteomyelitis are localized erythema, edema, pain, and lack of movement in the involved extremity. Management includes antibiotics and surgical drainage for joint infections (Gardner et al. 2020; Verklan et al. 2020).

Osteopenia is a decrease in the amount of calcium and phosphorus in the bone, which can lead to fractures. Risk factors include prematurity, diuretics, steroids, and lack of vitamin D. Signs of osteopenia are edema and limited mobility related to a fracture. Management includes supplementation and management of any fractures (Gardner et al. 2020; Verklan et al. 2020).

Resources
Merck Manual: New Ballard gestational age assessment tool: https://www.merckmanuals.com/professional/pediatrics/perinatal-problems/gestational-age

References

American Academy of Pediatrics & American Heart Association (2021) Textbook of neonatal resuscitation, 8th edn. American Academy of Pediatrics

Gardner SL, Carter BS, Enzman-Hines M, Niermeyer S (2020) Merenstein & Gardner's handbook of neonatal intensive care, 9th edn. Mosby Elsevier

Gleason C, Juul S (2018) Avery's diseases of the newborn, 10th edn. Elsevier

Kenner C, Altimier L, Boykova M, (eds.). (2019) Comprehensive neonatal nursing care, 6th edn. Springer Publishing Inc.

Lee H, Liu J, Profit J, Hintz S, Gould J (2020) Survival without major morbidity among very low birth weight neonates in California. Pediatrics 146(1):e20193865

Rogelet KR, Brorsen AJ (2016) Neonatal certification review for the CCRN and RNC high-risk examinations, 2nd edn, Jones & Bartlett Learning

Verklan M, Walden M, Forest S (eds) (2020) Core curriculum for neonatal intensive care, 6th edn. Elsevier

Predisposing and Contributing Factors for Nursing Errors

2

There are numerous factors that are involved with nursing errors and why they can occur. Errors should be viewed in terms of a "just culture," where the focus is on improving patient safety rather than blame. Just culture looks at accountability and faults within systems, rather than pointing fingers to blame one individual. When errors occur, processes often need improving or there is a lack of education. Just culture does not mean it is not a blame-free environment, and if there is an individual responsibility then that person must have accountability (Marx 2001; Maryniak 2019).

By using the just culture framework, incidents are reviewed based on duties rather than the outcome. Individual duties include a duty to produce an outcome, a duty to follow a procedural rule, and a duty to avoid unjustifiable risk. For a duty to produce an outcome, there are no specific procedures or steps in how to do something, but as an individual, it is expected that you will have a defined result. There may be an acceptable rate of failure for expectations. With a duty to follow a procedural rule, the expectation is that as an individual, we are expected to follow a procedure or policy in a specific way. The duty to avoid unjustifiable risk is described as an overarching duty for everyone. As individuals, generally, we do not do anything that is intentionally reckless; however, there are times when we may need to make a choice to do the right thing, but may breach and harm another value in the

K. Maryniak, *Controlling and Preventing Errors and Pitfalls in Neonatal Care Delivery*, https://doi.org/10.1007/978-3-031-25710-0_2

process; this is considered justifiable (Marx 2001; Maryniak 2019; Paradiso and Sweeney 2019; Rogers et al. 2017).

A breach of duty may occur for a variety of reasons, such as human error, at-risk behavior, and reckless behavior. Human error is an inadvertent action, or a slip, lapse, or mistake. In these circumstances a genuine mistake is made. A human error may include a skill-based mistake, an omission or forgetfulness, or a knowledge-based error (Marx 2001; Maryniak 2019). An example of a human error is a nurse who is drawing up a medication in the medication room and is interrupted. When she asks her co-worker to verify the dose, it is pointed out that she has drawn up the incorrect amount.

At-risk behavior is when someone chooses to do something that can inadvertently increase a chance for harm to occur. There is the potential for harm but it is not recognized by the person who is drifting away from consciously safer choices. The individual is aware that behavior is not following set practices, such as creating a work-around for a process. Many times, at-risk behaviors begin with system problems, such as ineffective processes, delays, or equipment problems. A work-around is found to deal with the system issue, but it creates behavior that becomes dangerous (Marx 2001; Maryniak 2019). One example of this is that there are not enough barcode scanners on a particular unit. As a workaround, to ensure medications are given on time, nurses begin to override the barcode scanning rather than waiting to use the scanner. This is a system problem (not enough barcode scanners), but the nurses have found a workaround which is an at-risk behavior.

With reckless behavior, an individual actually chooses an action that knowingly puts themselves or others in harm's way. The risk is identified but ignored. The individual is aware that their behavior is reckless, and there is a conscious disregard for others (Marx 2001; Maryniak 2019). One is example is a narcotic diversion. The nurse is aware that it is illegal but does not stop the behavior.

Repetitive errors with patient safety also need to be addressed. Even if it is a human error each time, repetitiveness indicates a deeper problem (Marx 2001; Maryniak 2019). An example is a nurse who has repeated medication errors. The root is determined to be human error with each event, yet there are still multiple occasions of the issue, which increases patient risk.

When looking at how nursing errors occur, it is important to understand which contributing factors are involved. Contributing factors are those that can cause an error or determine the level of risk, directly or indirectly. An error may be a result of one or a combination of contributing factors, which may be related to human, environmental, or organizational considerations.

Multiple studies have determined that human errors such as slips and lapses are the most common cause of nursing errors. Personal and environmental factors are frequently contributing causes of human errors. One condition that can lead to slips and lapses involves personal health status. This includes fatigue, sleep deprivation, and illness. Other physical signs, such as those indicating burnout, have been noted in studies which can be related to long hours and lack of breaks. Stress at work, lack of assertiveness, and personality also contributed to personal health. A busy work environment, distractions, interruptions, and pressure from others or time limitations can also increase the likelihood of human errors. Staff skill mix and workload are commonly identified as contributing to errors. This includes the volume of admissions, discharges, and transfers. Staffing with heavy patient loads and multitasking were other factors where omissions and violations occurred more often. Patient acuity was another condition identified as a contributing factor. This was particularly true when combined with other factors, often shown in medication errors of wrong time or dose omission. Studies have also demonstrated that short staffing is also a factor for errors, particularly when added to skill mix of staff, workload, and patient acuity (Donaldson et al. 2021; Roth et al. 2017).

Examples of slips and lapses involving medications include misidentifying either a medication or a patient. Contributing causes are misreading labels or documentation, look-a-like sound-a-like medications or patient names, lack of concentration, complacency, and carelessness. Further descriptions of errors will be covered in Chap. 3.

Knowledge-based mistakes were also noted in studies, but were less frequent. This included a lack of knowledge about disease processes, understanding about medications being administered or equipment that was being used, as well as unfamiliarity with the patient. Lack of critical thinking may be related to knowledge, personal, or environmental factors (Donaldson et al. 2021; Roth et al. 2017).

Written communication in studies included illegible and unclear documentation. Transcription errors also contributed to medication and procedure errors. These types of contributing factors were associated with facilities that still use written documentation or during downtime procedures. Other sources of inadequate written communication were a lack of appropriate policies, procedures, or protocols. Verbal communication, such as handoffs or interdisciplinary communications, was also noted in studies as contributing to errors (Krein et al. 2018; Roth et al. 2017).

Supplies and storage are also associated with errors. Logistics related to a unit or ward stock contributed to errors with medication and procedure times or omissions, including medication or supply misplacement. Delays in the delivery of medication or treatment, or unavailable medications and supplies were also sources of errors. Difficulties with equipment are another contributing condition to errors. Malfunctioning equipment, unfamiliarity or unclear equipment design, and insufficient availability of equipment contributed to errors (Donaldson et al. 2021; Krein et al. 2018).

Deliberate violations were not commonly seen in studies, and do not infer that there was malicious or ill intent. In these studies, violations were occurrences in which the nurses knew that processes were not followed, were situational, and were related to trusting colleagues, lack of appropriate protocols, patient acuity, and staff. The violations noted in studies related to medication errors were intentionally giving medications early or late, and administering medication without a signed order (Krein et al. 2018).

Reckless behaviors that lead to errors can include use of controlled substances at work, deliberately tampering with equipment or medications, or knowingly practicing outside of scope of practice. These types of behaviors are not typical but are dealt with through corrective action (Rogers et al. 2017).

References

Donaldson L, Ricciardi W, Sheridan S, Tartaglia R (eds) (2021) Textbook of patient safety and clinical risk management. Springer

Krein SL, Mayer J, Harrod M, Weston LE, Gregory L, Petersen L, Samore MH, Drews FA (2018) Identification and characterization of failures in infectious agent transmission precaution practices in hospitals: a qualitative study. JAMA Intern Med 178(8):1016–1057

Marx D (2001) Patient safety and the just culture: a primer for health care executives. Trustees of Columbia University, New York, NY

Maryniak K (2019) Professional nursing practice in the United States: an overview for international nurses, and those along the continuum from new graduates to experienced nurses

Paradiso L, Sweeney N (2019) Just culture. Nurs Manag 50(6):38–45

Rogers E, Griffin E, Carnie W, Melucci J, Weber RJ (2017) A just culture approach to managing medication errors. Hosp Pharm 52(4):308–315

Roth C, Brewer M, Wieck KL (2017) Using a Delphi method to identify human factors contributing to nursing errors. Nurs Forum 52(3):173–179

Types of Errors

Approximately 9.5% of all patient deaths annually in the United States are caused by medical errors (Institute of Medicine 2000; Johns Hopkins Medicine 2016), and that includes neonatal patients. It is difficult to quantify the statistics of medical errors with these vulnerable patients, but errors can include medication errors, delayed care, hospital-acquired infections, errors with equipment or devices, errors with procedures, and accidents, to name a few (ELMeneza and AbuShady 2020). Nurses play a key role in the prevention of errors, and unfortunately, they also play a key role in making errors. Many errors are due to poor processes or failure to follow policies and procedures.

Medical errors can be tragic in the NICU setting and rarely does a single problem or issue lead to an error. Good systems should have stable layers of defense against errors, but factors such as deviations from processes can cause a "Swiss cheese" effect which in turn leads to an error. System layers are at the point of patient care, individual healthcare professionals, the healthcare team, and the organization itself. Active failures in the system, latent conditions, human factors, and environmental hazards contribute to errors (Agency for Healthcare Research and Quality [AHRQ] 2019).

There are multiple common events that occur with neonates, and these unfortunate events can result in temporary or permanent harm, including death. Some common events are hospital-

© The Author(s), under exclusive license to Springer Nature Switzerland AG 2023
K. Maryniak, *Controlling and Preventing Errors and Pitfalls in Neonatal Care Delivery*, https://doi.org/10.1007/978-3-031-25710-0_3

acquired infections, adverse drug events, intravenous catheter extravasation, accidental extubation, and intracranial hemorrhage and ischemia. Other events include misidentification errors for medications, diagnostic tests, treatment, and documentation (Verklan et al. 2021).

Errors Associated with Hospital-Acquired Conditions

Although not all patient harm is associated with errors, some errors can result in hospital-acquired conditions. Nurses commonly perform what is referred to as "stacking," when there are multiple cognitive processes and competing priorities in the mind. The ability to manage many plans and thoughts for carrying out patient care through stacking can be impeded by the environment, changing situations, interruptions, delays, or time constraints. The practice environment consists of work design, adequate staffing, appropriate skill mix and assignments, organizational management, policies, resources, and the culture of the work environment (Al-ghraiybah et al. 2021; Thomas et al. 2017).

Hospital-acquired conditions (HACs) for neonatal patient include central line-associated bloodstream infections (CLABSIs), urinary tract infections (UTIs), ventilator-associated pneumonia (VAP), and hospital-acquired infections (also referred to as nosocomial infections). Healthcare-associated infections are also known as hospital-acquired infections or nosocomial infections. These infections are transmitted to the neonate in the environment, and may be caused by improper hand hygiene, invasive tubes and lines, peripheral lines, central lines, catheters, and ventilators. A CLABSI is a healthcare-associated infection, and risk factors are an increased risk with extended dwell time, improper sterile technique with insertion, dressing changes, poor hand hygiene, and open lines. The use of indwelling urinary catheters is not common with neonates, but a UTI, which may be another healthcare-associated infection, can occur. UTIs can cause bacteremia, meningitis, cystitis, and osteomyelitis. VAP is a healthcare-associated infection where pneumonia may be caused by Gram-positive or Gram-negative bacteria. Risk factors for VAP include prematurity, low birthweight, duration of ventilation, use of opiates, reintubation, frequent suctioning, enteral feeds, parenteral nutrition, steroids, and transfusion (Kenner et al. 2019).

Errors that can contribute to hospital-acquired conditions include a lack of appropriate or timely assessment. Assessment can be interrupted, delayed, or missed, due to the practice environment or issues affecting cognitive stacking (Al-ghraiybah et al. 2021; Roth et al. 2017; Thomas et al. 2017). Skin assessments are required frequently. Patients on ventilators should be assessed at least daily for continuation. Assessment of lines and drains is also necessary on a consistent basis. Missed assessments can lead to increased risk for CLABSIs and UTIs. Delayed or missing assessments of peripheral intravenous (IV) sites may also lead to infiltration or extravasation.

Delays, missed care opportunities, or not performing interventions can also occur, which are errors that can predispose patients to hospital-acquired conditions or falls (Al-ghraiybah et al. 2021; Roth et al. 2017; Thomas et al. 2017). Examples can be lack of perineal care or cleansing for patients with urinary catheter usage, which can lead to UTIs. Inappropriate cleaning of central line access can create an increased risk of CLABSIs. Failure to provide appropriate oral care can contribute to development of ventilator-associated pneumonia (VAP).

Failures in communication, both written and verbal, can also create errors (Roth et al. 2017; Thomas et al. 2017). Verbal communication mainly occurs with reports and handoffs. Using checklists and standardized tools to provide verbal communication can create more complete reports and ensure that vital patient information is passed along. Examples of communication tools may be SBAR or I-PASS (Miller 2021; Roth et al. 2017) (see also Chap. 6). Additionally, providing a bedside report with the off-going nurse, the oncoming nurse, and the family (if able) can ensure that there is a verbal and visual handoff, which can increase patient safety (Bigani and Correia 2018).

Complete documentation of assessment, interventions, and nursing care planning is essential. Assessments should be done real time, and documentation of lines and drains must be clear as well (Maryniak 2021). Even with complete documentation, nurses caring for patients must read what is charted and apply it. An important consideration to assist with critical thinking is looking for trends in patient care status. Identifying and applying trends is helpful in proactively planning and intervening on behalf of the patient (Maryniak 2021).

Errors Associated with the Environment and Developmental Care Needs

Neonates, as vulnerable patients, have additional considerations for the environment and developmental care needs. ELBW and VLBW neonates with serious complications, in particular, can result in significantly poor neurosensory outcomes such as neuro-motor problems and cognitive delays. The environment itself can negatively affect the growth and development of the neonate. Environmental considerations can include exposure to an extra-uterine environment, use of noisy technology, overwhelming light stimulation, and tactile sensations of touch and pain. These environmental stimuli can disrupt sleep and wake cycles and does not support premature brain growth. Additionally, interactions between caregivers and the neonate can also be impacted by the environment. Abrupt or inappropriate handling can disrupt the neonate's growth and development, and potentially increase the risk of IVH (Als and McAnulty 2015; Kenner et al. 2019).

Pain in the neonate can create physiological and behavioral outcomes and is not easily identified. The sympathetic nervous system of the neonate can have a decreased response to persistent and painful stimuli, which may obscure signs of pain or discomfort. General pain contributes to hypoxia, hypercarbia, acidosis, hyperglycemia, respiratory distress, and pneumothorax. Pain related to invasive procedures contribute to increased intrathoracic pressure, hypoxemic events, and alterations in oxygenation and cerebral volumes (Als and McAnulty 2015; Kenner et al. 2019). Strategies for providing developmentally appropriate care and pain management are essential in neonatal care.

Errors Related to Resuscitation

Some studies have identified errors related to neonatal resuscitation, including medication and procedural errors or delays. Lack of communication and teamwork can also create ineffective resuscitation which can create negative outcomes Errors in resuscitation have been estimated to occur at an average of 23% (Yamada et al. 2015). Resuscitation that is delayed or performed improperly can create lack of oxygen, resulting in brain injury and hypoxic-ischemic encephalopathy (ELMeneza and AbuShady 2020).

Neonatal resuscitation errors can include those of omission, which can cause negative clinical consequences that are significant. Examples of omission found in studies are failure to assess heart rate or breath sounds, or skipping steps within the resuscitation algorithm. Other errors are those with improper commission of steps or procedures, which are also associated with poor outcomes. Examples of commission errors are improper rates for giving ventilations or compression, poor positioning of bag and mask for ventilation, inadequate pressures with ventilation, incorrect technique for chest compression, and lack of synchronization of ventilations and compressions (Yamada et al. 2015).

Errors Associated with Medical Devices and Equipment

The use of equipment and medical devices is essential in caring for ill neonates, and occurs at a rate of 10–15%. Research studies show that intravenous infusion pumps and respiratory equipment were most commonly associated with equipment errors. Some consequences of errors with equipment or medical devices include inadequate or inappropriate ventilation, pneumothorax, atelectasis, skin integrity issues and damage, catheter occlusion, disruption of thermoregulation, and prolonged length of stay (Brado et al. 2021; ELMeneza et al. 2020).

Equipment malfunction can cause errors which may have significant effects on the neonates. Malfunctions can be from actual device failure, inadequate maintenance such as calibration, lack of technical support, equipment assembly issues, or poor equipment design. Lack of appropriate equipment is also associated with errors (Brado et al. 2021; ELMeneza et al. 2020).

Other causes of equipment or medical device errors are related to human factors. This includes distraction, fatigue, inadequate training, lack of experience, poor or unavailable policies and procedures, miscommunications, and time constraints (Brado et al. 2021; ELMeneza et al. 2020).

Errors Associated with Identification

Neonates are at a higher risk for identification errors as hospital bands may not be placed due to the fragility of skin. Techniques used with adult populations to confirm identities, such as verifying name and birthdate, cannot happen with neonatal populations. Studies have examined errors with neonates, including sentinel events, in which identification of the patient was a key factor. Errors associated with misidentification include procedural, medications, administration of breastmilk or formula, and incorrect laboratory or radiology results (Wallace 2016).

Errors Related to Procedures

There are multiple errors that can occur with procedures. The most common errors are mislabeled or unlabeled laboratory specimens and wrong patient reports. Failure to perform procedures correctly is another type of error, which can be the result of lack of knowledge or experience, time constraints, inappropriate or absent procedural standards, and environmental effects. Incorrect procedures can include vascular procedures such as the use of catheters, respiratory procedures, blood sampling, phototherapy, blood transfusion, and management of urinary catheters (El-Shazly et al. 2016; Wallace 2016).

Errors Affecting Skin Integrity

Neonates are at high risk for damage to the skin related to the immature integumentary system, and there are higher risks with premature and VLBW or ELBW neonates. Diligence is required to support skin integrity as a break in this first line of defense can easily create infection and sepsis in the neonate. Skin tears, epidermal stripping, and pressure injuries can occur. Skin injury from mechanical force is commonly seen in neonates, estimated at 40–45%. Medical devices contribute to skin injuries such as vascular catheters, respiratory equipment, and use of adhesives. Infiltration and extravasation are also seen in neonatal patients (August et al. 2021; ELMeneza et al. 2020).

Medication Errors

Medication errors that create patient harm are eight times more likely to occur in neonatal intensive care when compared to adult intensive care settings (Shawahna et al. 2022). It is difficult to quantify how many medication errors occur as there is no centralized reporting system for all errors. Some studies show that medication errors can occur between 32% and 94% of the time, with 38% of those errors attributed to nursing (Salar et al. 2020). Other studies specific to neonates demonstrated prescribing errors can be as high as 50%, and administration errors average 40% of the time (ELMeneza et al. 2020). The most common medication errors by nursing are wrong dose, wrong time, omissions, and wrong medication (MacDowell et al. 2021). Within the neonatal intensive care unit (NICU) setting, dosing errors are the most commonly reported medication errors (Shawahna et al. 2022).

Just as previously discussed, there are multiple contributing factors, which can lead to medication errors. Slips and lapses were identified in studies as a common cause of medication errors. Communications, supplies, and inadequate processes also contributed. Personal factors as well as system features can create a high risk for medication errors (Maryniak, 2016 and 2018).

Errors Related to Missed Nursing Care

Missed nursing care can lead to errors with neonates. Neonates can be cared for in a variety of settings, and there are many factors that can lead to missing nursing care opportunities. The most commonly found reasons cited in studies for missing nursing care are an emergency or deterioration of another patient. Studies discuss the most frequent areas of neonatal nursing care that are missed including providing developmental care, giving emotional support to parents, ensuring all important information is given during report, performing hand hygiene at all five moments of opportunity, providing skin care, assessing and cleaning eyes of neonates under phototherapy, and repositioning (Gathara et al. 2020; Kim and Chae 2022).

References

Agency for Healthcare Research and Quality (2019) Systems approach. https://psnet.ahrq.gov/primer/systems-approach

Al-ghraiybah T, Sim J, Lago L (2021) The relationship between the nursing practice environment and five nursing-sensitive patient outcomes in acute care hospitals: a systematic review. Nurs Open 8(5):2262–2271

Als H, McAnulty G (2015) Developmental care guidelines for use in the newborn intensive care unit (NICU). NIDCAP Federation International Web site http://www.inha.ie/wp-content/uploads/2015/07/INHA_ Developmental_Care_Guidelines.pdf

August D, Kandasamy Y, Ray R, Lindsay D, New K (2021) Fresh perspectives on hospital-acquired neonatal skin injury period prevalence from a multicenter study. J Perinat Neonatal Nurs 35(3):275–283

Bigani DK, Correia AM (2018) On the same page: nurse, patient, and family perceptions of change-of-shift bedside report. J Pediatr Nurs 41:84–89

Brado L, Tippmann S, Daniel S, Jonas J, Dorothea P et al (2021) Patterns of safety incidents in a neonatal intensive care unit. Frontiers in Pediatrics 9. https://doi.org/10.3389/fped.2021.664524/full

ELMeneza S, AbuShady M (2020) Anonymous reporting of medical errors from the Egyptian neonatal safety training network. Pediatr Neonatol 61(1):31–35

ELMeneza S, Elnaser A, Elmoean A, Elmoneem N (2020) Study of medical errors triggered by medical devices in neonatal intensive care unit. Edelweiss Pediatric Journal 1(1):7–12

El-Shazly A, Al-Azzouny M, Soliman D, Abed N, Attia S (2016) Medical errors in neonatal intensive care unit at Benha University Hospital, Egypt. Eastern Mediterranean Health Journal 23(1):31–39

Gathara D, Serem G, Murphy G, Obengo A, Tallam E et al (2020) Missed nursing care in newborn units: a cross-sectional direct observational study. BMJ Quality & Safety 29:19–30

Institute of Medicine (2000) To err is human: building a safer health system. National Academies Press, Washington (DC)

Johns Hopkins Medicine (2016) Study suggests medical errors now third leading cause of death in the U.S. https://www.hopkinsmedicine.org/news/media/releases

Kenner C, Altimier L, Boykova M (2019) Comprehensive neonatal nursing care, 6th edn. Springer Publishing Inc.

Kim S, Chae S (2022) Missed nursing care and its influencing factors among neonatal intensive care unit nurses: a descriptive study. Child Health Nursing Research 28(2):142–153

MacDowell P, Cabri A, Davis M (2021) Medication administration errors. Patient Safety Network https://psnet.ahrq.gov/primer/medication-administration-errors

Maryniak K (2016) How to avoid medication errors in nursing. https://www.rn.com/nursing-news/nurses-role-in-medication-error-prevention/

Maryniak K (2018) Medication errors: best practices for prevention (webinar). Lorman

Maryniak K (2021) Documentation for nurses, 4th edn. Elite Healthcare

Miller D (2021) I-PASS as a nursing communication tool. Pediatr Nurs 47(1):30–37

Roth C, Brewer M, Wieck KL (2017) Using a Delphi method to identify human factors contributing to nursing errors. Nurs Forum 52(3):173–179

Salar A, Kiani F, Rezaee N (2020) Preventing the medication errors in hospitals: a qualitative study. International Journal of Africa Nursing Sciences 13:100235

Shawahna R, Jaber M, Said R, Mohammad R, Aker Y (2022) Medication errors in neonatal intensive care units: a multicenter qualitative study in the Palestinian practice. BMC Pediatr 22:317

Thomas L, Donohue-Porter P, Fishbein J (2017) Impact of interruptions, distractions, and cognitive load on procedure failures and medication administration errors. J Nurs Care Qual 32(4):309–317

Verklan M, Walden M, Forest S (eds) (2021) Core curriculum for neonatal intensive care, 6th edn. Elsevier

Wallace S (2016) Newborns pose unique identification challenges. Pennsylvania Patient Safety Advisory 13(2):42–50

Yamada N, Yaeger K, Halamek L (2015) Analysis and classification of errors made by teams during neonatal resuscitation. Resuscitation 96:109–113

Consequences of Nursing Errors

4

Not all errors cause actual patient harm but there is a much higher risk of creating harm. Consequences related to errors have more detrimental effects on neonatal patients.

Levels of Harm

Nursing errors can be associated with a variety of patient outcomes. A near miss is when an error does not actually reach the patient but has the potential to cause harm. A near miss is an opportunity to identify a breakdown in the process before patient harm actually occurs (American Society for Healthcare Risk Management 2014; Maryniak 2018). One example of a near miss is a nurse who examines a syringe labeled for a dispensed single dose of intravenous metoclopramide. She sees that the syringe contains a solution that is cloudy. The nurse knows that IV metoclopramide should be clear. She does not give the medication, and reports the incident to pharmacy, returning the syringe that was dispensed.

No harm means that although an event reached a patient, there was no harm (American Society for Healthcare Risk Management 2014; Maryniak 2018). An illustration of an incident with no harm is a situation where an order for a neonatal patient is changed to increase oral feedings and decrease IV fluid rate. The nurse does not see the order at the time of the oral feeding and this change is not made immediately. Rather, the change in the volume of oral feedings and decreased IV fluids is made 3 h later. This is an error of delay, but there was no resulting harm to the patient.

Mild harm includes minimal symptoms or injury with minor interventions, observation, or increased length of stay (American Society for Healthcare Risk Management 2014; Maryniak 2018). An instance of mild harm is a new nurse who is still learning about handling neonatal patients with developmentally supportive strategies. He is preparing to weigh the patient on the warmer and lifts the neonate off the warmer to zero on the scale. He does not contain the neonate, and when lifted the neonate demonstrates an abrupt startle reflex, with splaying and grimacing. The neonate is placed back on the warmer for the weight, and continues to show distressing behavior as well as desaturations, tachypnea, and tachycardia, followed by a brief episode of apnea and bradycardia. When the patient is repositioned and contained, vital signs return to baseline and the patient's behaviors become relaxed. Although there was initial harm, there was no lasting harm.

Moderate harm means that the patient has a bodily or psychological injury which affects quality of life or function (American Society for Healthcare Risk Management 2014; Maryniak 2018). An example is a nurse who does not perform blood sampling via a heel stick appropriately. She uses a lancet that is too big for the patient's size, and punctures deeply near the heel. Nurses assess the site, which becomes reddened, swollen, and painful to the patient. The patient develops osteomyelitis, confirmed by testing. Management includes antibiotics, wound care, and minimal handling. This is moderate harm as there was patient injury that affected the patient's quality of life and additional treatment which potentially increased the length of stay. The neonate recovers from the infection without apparent long-term consequences.

Severe harm indicates physical or psychological injury to a patient, which significantly affects function or quality of life (American Society for Healthcare Risk Management 2014; Maryniak 2018). One case of severe harm is a patient who had extravasation from a peripheral infusion of TPN located in the right hand. The incident happened during a very busy shift in the

NICU, and the nurse did not assess the IV site for several hours. When she checked the site, it was blistering and discolored, and the hand and arm were cold and severely swollen. She immediately removed the cannula, attempted aspiration, and gave hyaluronidase per provider's order. The hand and part of the arm became necrotic, and a plastic surgeon was consulted. It was determined that plastic surgery was warranted, and there was a high likelihood that future mobility of the hand and arm would be impacted. The harm was severe, with significant effects on the patient's quality of life.

Death is the last patient outcome as a result of an event (American Society for Healthcare Risk Management 2014; Maryniak 2018). Some well-known examples, unfortunately, were heparin overdoses that occurred in NICUs. There have been incidents where heparin was available in strengths up to 10,000 units/mL. Errors occurred from either inadvertently mixing inappropriately, dispensing incorrectly or having wrong doses available, and administration of incorrect concentrations, leading to overdoses. In these cases, multiple neonates died from these errors.

Avoidable Harm

Errors related to the care of neonates cannot only harm one patient, but can possibly harm others. Failure to perform hand hygiene or use PPE appropriately can increase the risk of exposure to the healthcare professional through contamination. This in turn can put the caregiver at risk, as well as increased risk of spreading infectious diseases to other patients. A higher chance of contagion spread to other patients or even loved ones of the healthcare professional at home may occur (Fan et al. 2020). Examples include the spread of MDROs in a hospital setting, such as MRSA in a neonatal intensive care unit (NICU). MRSA can often be spread by individuals who are colonized with the bacteria, usually from a community-acquired setting. Many studies have shown that outbreaks in a NICU setting can be traced to a healthcare professional who unknowingly passes along MRSA to these vulnerable patients (Brown et al. 2019; Huang et al. 2019; Popoola et al. 2014). Diligent hand hygiene and appropriate use of PPE can help prevent these outbreaks, along with other strategies.

Avoidable patient harm that can occur from errors can also increase morbidity and mortality. Both short- and long-term effects may be seen. Hospital-acquired conditions such as CLABSIs, UTIs, VAP, pressure injuries, and other hospital-acquired infections can cause unnecessary patient pain and suffering, complex conditions, potential disability, and impact on both physical and psychological states. Other consequences include longer lengths of stay (and all of the associated risks with that), as well as increased costs to the healthcare system (Panagioti et al. 2019).

Harmful Effects on Growth and Development

Care for neonatal patients can increase harmful effects on the growth and development. IVH is one condition that can be caused without diligent care, particularly with extreme prematurity and ELBW infants. Hemodynamic instability can cause IVH, such as hypotension or hypertension, and the use of bolus fluids. Disruptions in homeostasis such as hyperosmolality, hyperglycemia, hypoglycemia, and acid–base imbalances also increase the risk for IVH. Inappropriate positioning, abrupt handling, and environmental stimuli also have negative effects including a higher possibility for IVH (Rogelet and Brorsen 2016).

Other long-term complications are seen with neonates that can be influenced by errors in handling and care, especially in those populations of premature, VLBW, and ELBW infants. For example, there is a higher incidence of developing cerebral palsy. Poor neurosensory outcomes such as emotional and behavioral problems can occur. Long-term sleep difficulties may happen. Behavioral problems may include hyperactivity, attention deficit, and depression (Rogelet and Brorsen 2016).

Central-Line-Associated Bloodstream Infections

A CLABSI is a central-line-associated bloodstream infection. The most vulnerable patients for developing CLABSIs include neonatal intensive care patients due to the high utilization rates of central lines. CLABSI rates for all populations have been 4.1–5.3 cases per 1000 patient line days internationally (Agency for Healthcare Research and Quality 2020; Asia Pacific Society of Infection Control 2015). Within neonatal populations, CLABSI rates range from 2.35 to 8.62 cases per 1000 patient line days, with the highest rates in ELBW patients (Schmid et al. 2018). CLABSI is associated with high mortality and morbidity among healthcare-acquired infections, due to bacteremia or fungal invasion, at a rate of 20,000–30,000 people each year (Agency for Healthcare Research and Quality [AHRQ] 2020; Asia Pacific Society of Infection Control 2015). Excess mortality examines additional deaths that are directly related to an infectious HAC. One meta-analysis that was done on all patient populations estimated that there are 150 excess deaths per 1000 cases of CLABSI, which is a rate of 0.15 (AHRQ 2017). Even in situations where there is no patient death, developing a CLABSI can cause the neonatal patient pain and stress.

Urinary Tract Infections

A UTI is a urinary tract infection, and neonatal patients are vulnerable to developing a UTI when there is a use of urinary catheters. UTIs commonly occur with neonatal patients, and rates can be as high as 25% of patients in the NICU (Aviles-Otero et al. 2020; Gorski et al. 2021). Most neonatal UTIs are from *E. coli*. Risks for UTIs are prematurity, comorbidities, VLBW and ELBW, female gender, and urinary catheterization. Developing a UTI can be painful and create other patient complications, including sepsis.

Ventilator-Associated Pneumonia

Ventilator-associated events (VAEs) are those that cause deterioration in respiratory status after a period of stability or improvement on the ventilator, with evidence of infection or inflammation, and laboratory evidence of respiratory infection. Ventilator-associated pneumonia (VAP) is one form of VAE, and is the common hospital-acquired infection in intensive care units. VAP rates in NICUs range from 2.7 to 10.9 cases per 1000 ventilator days (Goerens et al. 2018). The length of time for intubation is a risk factor, and studies estimate up to 20% of critically ill neonates develop VAP after 48 h of intubation (Wang et al. 2021). VAP is associated with long-term outcomes including chronic lung disease as well as neonatal mortality, with mortality rates as high as 16% (Wang et al. 2021).

Disruption of Skin Integrity

Pressure injuries are those that cause localized injury to the skin and underlying tissue. These injuries may or may not be pressure ulcers, and are generally seen over a bony prominence. Pressure injuries are caused by pressure and shear, or a combination of both. Neonates are vulnerable due to premature skin, lack of subcutaneous fat, limited mobility, disease processes, incontinence, and use of devices and adhesives. Studies of skin injury in neonatal patients estimate the prevalence as 9–43% (Broom et al. 2019). Neonatal skin injury significantly increases the risk of developing infections and sepsis (Araújo et al. 2022).

Medication Errors

Medication errors can range in patient harm from near misses to patient death. Studies of NICU settings estimate medication error rates between 4 and 35.1 per 1000 patient-days, and between 5.5 and 77.9 per 100 medication orders. Dosing errors are the most commonly reported medication errors in neonatal patients (Shawahna et al. 2022). In addition to incorrect doses, other recurrent medication errors with neonatal patients include dose omission, wrong route of administration, wrong intervals between medications, and medication administration after discontinuation by a provider (Eslami et al. 2019).

Medication errors may also cause adverse drug events (ADEs), which are often associated with patient harm. Errors associated with high-risk medications are those that often lead to severe harm, disability, or even death. Preventable patient injury from medication errors, although not common, can have a long-term impact on the patient and family (Afreen et al. 2021).

An ADE is harm that occurs as a result of a medication. Not all ADEs are result of an error. For example, heparin-induced thrombocytopenia (HIT) is a reaction that occurs from the use of heparin. HIT is considered an ADE, even when the medication is administered appropriately. A preventable ADE is one that is associated with a medication error which causes patient harm. It is estimated that about 5% of all hospitalized patients experience a preventable ADE (PSNet 2019). Risk factors for an ADE in hospital are neonatal and pediatric patients, polypharmacy, high-alert medications, use of look-alike, sound-alike medications, and ineffective processes or non-compliance with safe medication administration (PSNet 2019). Excess mortality is estimated at 0.012, or 12 excess deaths for every 1000 ADEs (AHRQ 2017).

Widespread Effects of Patient Harm

Errors that occur in healthcare can also have effects on others. Trust between the family and the healthcare team can be negatively affected by an error. This can occur even if there is disclosure about the error, although the impact on the family's perception may be improved with disclosure. The Institute of Medicine's report, *To Err is Human* (1999), states most errors are systemic but often decrease trust in the healthcare professional who made the error. Institutions that are not proactive, transparent, or create action when an error occurs can cause a patient to feel betrayed.

This betrayal is often directed at the healthcare professional, rather than being at the organization that had systemic issues (Smith 2017). Families who have neonatal patients, particularly those who are sick and critically ill, are in a state of crisis. They may be experiencing grief, fear, and life stress from the situation alone. Errors in the care of their baby can exacerbate these emotions even if there is no patient harm. And if errors cause neonatal harm or even death, these events are significantly intensified, with long-term effects on the family members as well as the patients.

The healthcare professional themselves may also be impacted by an error. Second victim syndrome is a term for the healthcare professional, such as a nurse, who has committed an error. The professional feel responsible, particularly if the error is associated with a poor outcome. The person may feel shame, guilt, anxiety, grief, depression, compassion dissatisfaction, burnout, secondary traumatic stress, and physical manifestations. The psychological effects are not just about responsibility, but go deeper to where the healthcare professional can be traumatized as a result of the event (Ozeke et al. 2019).

Nursing errors can also impact the organization itself. Patient harm resulting from errors has financial effects. There are higher costs associated with longer lengths of stay. And hospital-acquired conditions are not reimbursed by insurance companies. The additional costs for a patient who develops a CLABSI is an average of $48,000 US dollars, with a range of $27,000 to $69,000 (AHRQ 2017). VAP has an average cost of $47,000 with a range of $22,000 to $72,000 (AHRQ 2017). Neonatal sepsis cost up to $129,000 per case, many of which are results of hospital-acquired infection (Salman et al. 2020). Additional costs for ADEs are estimated at $5800, ranging from $4000 to $15,000 (AHRQ 2017).

Additionally, there may be lawsuits against an organization for patient harm that is caused by error. The lawsuits themselves can cost an organization financially, but the public perception of the organization may also be affected. Long-term, the organization's reputation may be damaged which can lead to further negative financial impact (Adler et al. 2018).

References

Adler L, Yi D, Li M, McBroom B, Hauck L et al (2018) Impact of inpatient harms on hospital finances and patient clinical outcomes. J Patient Saf 14(2):67–73

Afreen N, Padilla-Tolentino E, McGinnis B (2021) Identifying potential high-risk medication errors using telepharmacy and a web-based survey tool. Innovations in Pharmacy 12(1):10

Agency for Healthcare Research and Quality (AHRQ) (2017) Estimating the additional hospital inpatient cost and mortality associated with selected hospital-acquired conditions. https://www.ahrq.gov/hai/pfp/haccost2017-results.html

Agency for Healthcare Research and Quality (AHRQ) (2020) Guide: purpose and use of CLABSI tools. https://www.ahrq.gov/hai/clabsi-tools/guide.html

American Society for Healthcare Risk Management (2014) Serious safety events: a focus on harm classification: deviation in care as link. http://www.ashrm.org/pubs/files/white_papers/SSE-2_getting_to_zero-9-30-14.pdf

Araújo D, Araújo J, Silva A, Lopes J, Dantas A, Martins Q (2022) Alteration of skin condition in newborns admitted to neonatal intensive care: a concept analysis. Rev Bras Enfermary 75(4):e20210473

Asia Pacific Society of Infection Control (2015) APSIC guide for prevention of central line associated bloodstream infections (CLABSI). https://apsic-apac.org/wp-content/uploads/2016/09/APSIC-CLABSI-guidelines-FINAL-20-Jan-2015.pdf

Aviles-Otero N, Ransom M, Sullivan B, Charlton J, Hendrik Weitkamp J, Fairchild K, Kaufman D (2020) Abnormal heart rate characteristics predict urinary tract infections in VLBW infants. Pediatrics 146(1_MeetingAbstract):370–372

Broom M, Dunk AM, Mohamed E (2019) Predicting neonatal skin injury: the first step to reducing skin injuries in neonates. Health Service Insights 14:12

Brown N, Reacher M, Rice W, Roddick I, Reeve L et al (2019) An outbreak of methicillin-resistant staphylococcus aureus colonization in a neonatal intensive care unit: use of a case-control study to investigate and control it and lessons learnt. Journal of Hospital Infections 103(1):35–43

Eslami K, Aletayeb F, Aletayeb S, Kouti L, Hardani A (2019) Identifying medication errors in neonatal intensive care units: a two-center study. BMC Pediatr 19(1):365

Fan J, Jiang Y, Hu K, Chen X, Xu Q et al (2020) Barriers to using personal protective equipment by healthcare staff during the COVID-19 outbreak in China. Medicine 99(48):e23310

Goerens A, Lehnick D, Büttcher M, Daetwyler K, Fontana M et al (2018) Neonatal ventilator associated pneumonia: a quality improvement initiative focusing on antimicrobial stewardship. Front Pediatr 24(6):262

Gorski D, Bauer A, Menda N, Hareraniel M (2021) Treatment of positive urine cultures in the neonatal intensive care unit: a guideline to reduce antibiotic utilization. J Perinatol 41(6):1474

Huang H, Ran J, Yang J, Li P, Zhuang G (2019) Impact of MRSA transmission and infection in a neonatal intensive care unit in China: a bundle intervention study during 2014–2017. BioMed Research International. https://www.hindawi.com/journals/bmri/2019/5490413/

Institute of Medicine (1999) To err is human: building a safer health system. National Academy Press

Maryniak K (2018) Medication errors: best practices for prevention (webinar). Lorman

Ozeke O, Ozeke V, Coskun O, Budakoglu II (2019) Second victims in health care: current perspectives. Adv Med Educ Pract 10:593–603

Panagioti M, Khan K, Keers R, Abuzour A, Phipps D et al (2019) Prevalence, severity, and nature of preventable patient harm across medical care settings: systematic review and meta-analysis. BMJ 366:l4185

Popoola V, Budd A, Wittig S, Ross T, Aucott S et al (2014) Methicillin-resistant staphylococcus aureus transmission and infections in a neonatal intensive care unit despite active surveillance cultures and decolonization: challenges for infection prevention. Infect Control Hosp Epidemiol 35(4):412–418

PSNet (2019) Medication errors and adverse drug events. https://psnet.ahrq.gov/primer/medication-errors-and-adverse-drug-events

Rogelet KR, Brorsen AJ (2016) Neonatal certification review for the CCRN and RNC high-risk examinations, 2nd edn, Jones & Bartlett Learning

Salman O, Procter S, McGregor C, Paul P, Hutubessy R, Lawn J, Jit M (2020) Systematic review on the acute cost-of-illness of sepsis and meningitis in neonates and infants. Pediatr Infect Dis J 39(1):35–40

Schmid S, Geffers C, Wagenpfeil G, Simon A (2018) Preventive bundles to reduce catheter-associated bloodstream infections in neonatal intensive care. GMS Hygiene & Infection Control 16:13

Shawahna R, Jaber M, Said R, Mohammad R, Aker Y (2022) Medication errors in neonatal intensive care units: a multicenter qualitative study in the Palestinian practice. BMC Pediatr 22:317

Smith C (2017) First, do no harm: institutional betrayal and trust in health care organizations. J Multidiscip Healthc 10:133–144

Wang H, Tsai M, Chu S, Liao C, Lai M et al (2021) Clinical characteristics and outcomes of neonates with polymicrobial ventilator-associated pneumonia in the intensive care unit. BMC Infect Dis 21:965

Monitoring for and Detecting Nursing Errors

Identifying errors can be difficult and time consuming. Most facilities have an event reporting system that is used to track and trend events once identified. It is more concerning that there are errors that go undetected or unreported due to fear of reprisal or punishment. It is important for facilities to adopt a safety program that is non-punitive to encourage event reporting, a culture of open communication, transparency, and a quality assurance program that proactively monitors for abnormalities. Facilities should also have a strong internal audit program, including proactive risk assessments to help identify errors that may not be reported.

Nurses spend the majority of their time documenting, and sometimes there is the thought that outcomes are improved through the act of documentation itself. Documentation is part of the process but should not be used to control a process. Nurses feel frustrated and overwhelmed with overcomplicated documentation that takes time away from the patient. Documentation should help guide the nurse but not be overly burdensome (Maryniak 2021). Nurses need to spend their critical thinking skills on patient assessment and needs, not on remembering all the nuances of documentation requirements.

Documentation should direct the nurse in telling the patient's story in a way that the next caregivers understand what they need to provide good care (Maryniak 2021). If nurses are struggling with documentation, then assessment of how the nursing

© The Author(s), under exclusive license to Springer Nature Switzerland AG 2023
K. Maryniak, *Controlling and Preventing Errors and Pitfalls in Neonatal Care Delivery*, https://doi.org/10.1007/978-3-031-25710-0_5

documentation is set up must be done. The question should be asked if the documentation is set up in a way that helps guide the nurse to be successful and gives the appropriate information. If there are a lot of documentation errors or handoff events, the documentation templates should be examined.

A root cause analysis (RCA) is a process of working toward discovering the real cause of a problem. The focus is on resolving the actual cause, rather than just looking at the symptoms of the issue. Contributing factors are identified during discussion of the event. An RCA does not need to be done with every problem, as it is a time-consuming process. However, there are times when an RCA is required, such as with serious safety events (e.g., never events or severe patient harm), repeat safety events, reportable patient injury (e.g., hospital-acquired conditions), a near miss with high potential for harm, family complaints, and at the discretion of leadership.

One method of analysis for an RCA is where a team looks at five "whys." In this method, the question "why" is asked repeatedly until the original reason for the error, also known as the root cause of a problem, is found (Maryniak 2019) (see also Fig. 5.1). A visual diagram, such as a fishbone, may be a useful tool to depict the contributing factors (see Fig. 5.2). Alternatively, the data about contributing factors from the RCA discussion can be listed in a Table (see Fig. 5.3).

Many staff and leaders have been involved in root cause analysis or improvement plans. Following an RCA, a plan of corrective action should be developed. These plans should include measurable and effective goals. An example of a table used for corrective

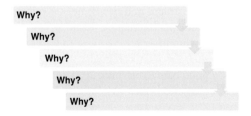

Fig. 5.1 Example of the "five why's"

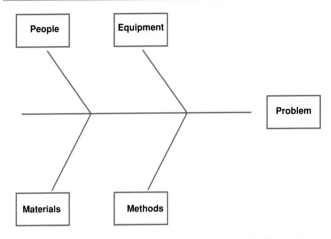

Fig. 5.2 Example of a fishbone diagram. Maryniak (2019). *Professional nursing practice in the United States: An overview for international nurses, and those along the continuum from new graduates to experienced nurses.* Author. (Used with permission)

Category	Contributing Factors
People	
Processes	
Equipment, supplies	
Culture	
Communication	
Staffing, training	

Fig. 5.3 Example of contributing factors table

action is in Fig. 5.4. The key to making and sustaining actual improvement from an RCA is to determine goals and actions that are reasonable, actionable, and valuable.

Where there are errors, many times the first suggestions are to provide education and add some form of documentation audit. Those strategies are not generally effective, especially if the

Corrective Action	Measure of Success	Responsible Party	Due to Review

Fig. 5.4 Corrective action planning table

investigation and strategies do not get to the root cause of the error. And usually, the audits are given to the nurses to perform, which takes away time spent with patients. To address issues and assist nurses the processes and workspaces must be examined. Wastes must be reduced or eliminated from processes to help improve outcomes. Examples of waste can include time spent searching for supplies, over-documentation, visual clutter, and constant interruptions. There is a term called "value added" in Lean Six Sigma for process steps (Sweeney 2016). If a step does not add value, cannot be done right the first time, and is not something the customer is willing to pay for then that step should be eliminated if possible.

If there are multiple errors found in a process that have different root causes, a good consideration would be to complete a Failure Modes and Effects Analysis (FMEA) to assess for vulnerability in the process. An FMEA can help identify vulnerable process steps, prioritize them by risk stratification, and implement mitigation strategies to decrease or eliminate the vulnerability (see also Fig. 5.5).

A culture of transparency and open communication is important to increase safety and decrease errors. This does not just happen; it must be planned and groomed. Many organizations that adopt lean principles use a type of daily management system to ensure open communication between frontline staff and leadership. This can be as simple as a whiteboard used to communicate frontline needs and leadership expectations. Criteria is established to note and communicate the conditions for the shift, if there needs to be adjustments to workflow due to call offs, number of patients in isolation, if there is equipment unavailable so staff are

Failure Modes and Effects Analysis (FMEA) Form

Process/Product Name:

Problem:

Prepared by:

FMEA Date:

Severity (SEV): How severe is the effect on the customer? (5- most severe; 1- least severe)

Probability of Occurrence (OCC): How often does the cause occur? (5= highest occurrence; 1= lowest occurrence)

Detectability (DET): How well can you detect of the cause using the current controls? (5=most difficult to detect; 1= easily detected)

Risk Priority Number (RPN): What is the measure of process risk related to the effects, causes, & controls? (RPN + OCC+ DET)

Process Step/Input	Potential Failure Mode	Potential Failure Effects	SEV	Potential Causes	OCC	Current Controls	DET	RPN	Action Recommended	Responsibility	Follow Up: Actions Taken	Final SEV	Final OCC	Final DET	Final RPN
What is the process step under investigation?	What can go wrong with the process step/output?	What is the impact on the customer or internal requirements?		What are the root cause reasons for the process step/output to go wrong?		What are the existing controls that prevent or detect either the cause prior to leaving the process step?			What are the actions for reducing the OCC of the cause?	What is the target completion date and who is responsible?	What actions were completed and when?				
								0							0
								0							0
								0							0
								0							0
								0							0

Fig. 5.5 Example of an FMEA form

aware, etc. Leaders can use the board to help guide their rounding and to alert staff to new processes or process changes. The purpose is to improve the safety and quality of care for patients by ensuring that those who care for the patients are well equipped, those who lead the caregivers are well informed, and ensure a connection to purpose.

An example of a daily management board includes the following information:

- Census, number of patients in isolation.
- Staffing available for the shift and on-call staff.
- Supplies that are on backorder, broken or missing equipment, and estimated time available.
- Identification of high-risk patients.
- New process, change in the current process.

The caregivers can be better prepared for the shift and aware of the department's issues. The leaders can use the information to prioritize their rounding and monitor high-risk patients in the department. Leaders can have a bigger impact on safety if they assist in real-time monitoring of high-risk patients and processes instead of the status quo of retrospective monitoring. Real time, concurrent monitoring with immediate feedback is more effective in process control and connecting the purpose (the "why") than retrospective monitoring. If problems are found days, weeks, or months after the fact they are much harder to correct.

Using concurrent monitoring and mentoring can have an impact on the majority of healthcare-associated infections and accidents. It is known that with each day a neonate is intubated or has a central line in place the chance of infection increases. Tightly controlled use of devices can decrease infection rates substantially. Education should focus on the dangers of using devices when they are not medically necessary, and why it is important to remove these as soon as possible (Letica-Kriegel et al. 2019). The daily management board can alert nurses and leaders of the patients in the department with these devices to increase attention to care and removal of the devices. Charge nurses can assess if the

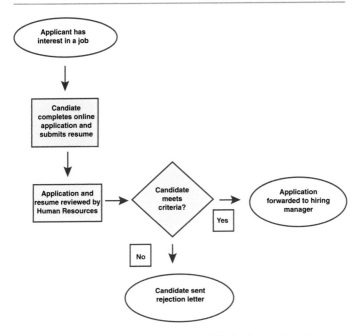

Fig. 5.6 Example of flowchart. Maryniak (2019). *Professional nursing practice in the United States: An overview for international nurses, and those along the continuum from new graduates to experienced nurses.* Author (Used with permission)

device is medically necessary and the leader can assess that the care is appropriate, providing real-time feedback to caregivers present of any deviations noted. The old saying "it takes a village" applies to patient safety. It takes the entire team to keep patients safe. Tools such as a flowchart or value stream map can be useful to look at and evaluate the current state, and determine future state (see Figs. 5.6 and 5.7).

The only way a nurse leader can assess what their nurses are spending their time doing is by monitoring them where the work is happening. In Lean Six Sigma this is called going to the Gemba—going to where the work happens (Sweeney 2016). It is the responsibility of nursing leadership to provide the tools and

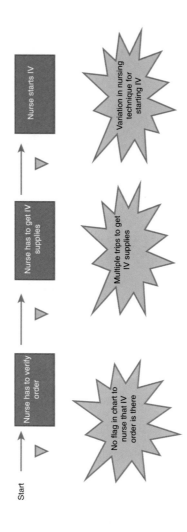

Fig. 5.7 Example of value stream analysis. Maryniak (2019). *Professional nursing practice in the United States: An overview for international nurses, and those along the continuum from new graduates to experienced nurses.* Author (Used with permission)

resources the nurse needs to provide a high-quality patient care. The only way to truly assess this is by going to where the work is being done and watching, asking questions, and seeing what works and what does not work.

An example of going to the Gemba occurred at a facility to help reduce medication errors in a level II special care nursery. When reviewing the events, it was noted that there was a high number of errors at a specific time of the day. Observations were made during that time period to watch the medication pass within the unit. It was demonstrated that nurses were interrupted more than 30 times total at the automated dispensing unit. There was an immediate review of the medication records, and several missed or delayed doses were found. This information was provided to the department director, and the location of the automated dispensing unit for this department was changed. This in turn led to a decrease in medication errors by over 50%. The nurses did not realize they were interrupted so often because they were so used to getting disrupted. The observations and outcomes brought more awareness to the director and the nurses. Therefore, it is important for leaders to go where the work is and watch. The caregivers do not always recognize the contributing factors to errors because they develop a bias toward them. Having fresh eyes on a situation can help find contributing factors that can be mitigated or even eliminated.

Standard work is also important to ensure that all caregivers complete processes the same and the outcomes are predictable. It would be very difficult to monitor a process if there is no standard way agreed on to complete the process. There are best practices available for many of the safety protocols, including monitoring and documentation. There should be standard expectations for the care of high-risk patient types that can be monitored easily by leadership. An example going back to indwelling central lines includes monitoring the care bundle. The caregivers should be aware of the best practices in caring for patients with central lines, including bundle elements for line insertion and maintenance. This information should be easy to understand and simple to monitor. If a process is not written down, it is not standard work.

Another concept of lean principles is mutual respect. Leaders are responsible for leading by example, managing their peers and staff in a way that builds mutual respect. This further improves the culture of safety in facilities which is imperative for patient safety and high-quality of care. When a leader focuses on processes and does not blame caregivers immediately for errors, caregivers are more likely to report errors because they feel safe to do so. Transparency is a two-way street when it comes to safety and high reliability. If the leaders make promises, it should be transparent to staff so they are held accountable for their actions as well.

Planning is essential, and considerations include the communication plan from frontline caregivers to leaders and vice versa. Another consideration is how errors are handled, and does the organization cultivate a culture of blame or does it look for cause, contributing factors, and process issues. Caregivers should know what is expected of them, and the leader's expectations must be clear with a connection to purpose. The organization needs to identify high-risk patients in departments, and staff must work as a team to care for these patients and ensure they are not further compromised. Processes should be easy to find and must be written in a way that all of the caregivers understand and follow them. Workarounds are due to poor processes or obstacles that continue to cause barriers and must be identified to make process improvements.

Other strategies to monitor for nursing errors include interdisciplinary rounding and leader rounding. Interdisciplinary rounding is valuable for nursing staff to ensure patient needs are met, which contributes to patient safety. Rounding on patients by nursing leaders is also helpful to focus on patient safety. Examples with neonates include ensuring bundles are in compliance (such as central line bundles), assessment of IV sites, and ensuring developmental care needs are met, such as environmental stimuli and supportive positioning (Maryniak 2019).

Bedside nurses are also essential in identifying potential and actual errors. Catching errors before they occur or recognizing areas of opportunity with policies, procedures, and protocols can make differences in current practices. With the increase in comorbidities and infections, it is important that nurses use tools to improve communication, transparency, and ensure the work is standardized and easily accessible and understood.

References

Letica-Kriegel AS, Salmasian H, Vawdrey DK, Youngerman BE, Green RA, Furuya EY, Calfee DP, Perotte R (2019) Identifying the risk factors for catheter-associated urinary tract infections: a large cross-sectional study of six hospitals. BMJ Open 9(2):e022137

Maryniak K (2019) Professional nursing practice in the United States: an overview for international nurses, and those along the continuum from new graduates to experienced nurses.

Maryniak K (2021) Documentation for nurses, 4th edn. Elite Healthcare

Sweeney B (2016) Lean six sigma quickstart guide: the simplified beginner's guide to lean six sigma, ClydeBank Media

Best Practices to Prevent Nursing Errors

6

Scope of Practice

When looking at the potential for errors, nurses need to consider what is included in their nursing scope of practice. Scope of practice determines the limitations and accountabilities of nurses. Although nursing scope of practice varies by location (such as state or province of licensure), there are some general common considerations included within scope of practice. It is essential that nurses understand his or her scope of practice within their geographic location (e.g., state or province) (Maryniak 2019).

Examples of limitations within nursing scope of practice are that a nurse can only administer medications that are ordered by a licensed provider; nurses cannot order medications. A provider may order protocols that identify specific circumstances and parameters for medication administration. Protocols may be implemented within an organization that define circumstances or parameters for medication administration. One example of a protocol that may be seen with neonatal patients is for narcotic withdrawal management. Neonatal abstinence syndrome (NAS) has management strategies that include non-pharmacological and pharmacological. Providers may have medication dosing associated with patient scoring on a NAS tool Another practice consideration is that it is also beyond the scope of the nurse to medically diagnose (Maryniak 2019).

© The Author(s), under exclusive license to Springer Nature Switzerland AG 2023
K. Maryniak, *Controlling and Preventing Errors and Pitfalls in Neonatal Care Delivery*, https://doi.org/10.1007/978-3-031-25710-0_6

Nursing accountabilities within scope of practice include that actions and interventions based on nursing assessment must either be ordered or be included in policies, procedures, and protocols. This includes interventions that are part of medication administration. Nursing accountabilities include assessment, recognizing patient status changes, and using nursing judgment (Maryniak 2019).

Bedside Report

Bedside report, also known as shift report or nursing handoff, is another effective strategy to help prevent errors. With bedside report, both the oncoming and offgoing nurses participate in handoff at the bedside of the patient. The goal is to include the family in the report, which helps improve communication between staff and family. Research has shown that communication breakdown is correlated with adverse events (AHRQ, n.d.). Studies have also shown that bedside reporting increases family satisfaction, and does improve nursing satisfaction as well, when it is done effectively (Dorvil 2018; Maryniak 2019). Standardized bedside reports can focus on safety, such as double checks with patient lines and equipment, activities, and plan of care. This interactive report can also assist in reinforcing family teaching (AHRQ n.d.; Maryniak 2019).

A recommended process for bedside report is as follows:

- Introduce the nursing staff to the family (if present), and invite them to participate in the bedside report.
- Access the health record.
- The off-going nurse will conduct a verbal report with the oncoming nurse and family (see Standardized Communication section below).
- Use words that the family can understand.
- The oncoming nurse will conduct a safety inspection of the room, and a focused assessment of the patient.
  - Visually inspect all IV sites and tubing, wounds, etc.
  - Visually sweep the area for any physical safety concerns.

- Both nurses will review tasks that were done, or need to be done, such as:
  - Labs or tests needed.
  - Medications administered.
- Identify the patient's needs and family's needs or concerns, and discuss the goal(s).
- Some questions to ask the family may include:
  - "What could have gone better (during the shift)?"
  - "What concerns do you have?"
  - "What do you want to happen (during the next shift)?"
- Follow up to see if the goal was met during the next bedside report.

  (AHRQ n.d.)

Interdisciplinary Rounding

Rounding with neonatal patients looks very different than in the adult inpatient world, where purposeful patient rounding is routinely performed. Neonatal patient needs include regular safety checks, such as ensuring equipment is working appropriately, IV sites are assessed, patient comfort and positioning is assessed, and families are included. In addition to these basic needs, interdisciplinary rounding for bedside rounds is a best practice. Rounds at the bedside allow multiple disciplines to participate in reviewing patients and decision-making about care. Family members should also be included in bedside rounds when possible, which increases their participation and improves transparency and communication. Studies have shown that interdisciplinary rounds increase patient safety as well as improve staff and family satisfaction rates (Cham et al. 2021; Shivananda et al. 2022).

A great interdisciplinary team requires respect, understanding of everyone's role, and effective communication. A team focus in addition to flexibility and vision assists with quality outcomes. The culture and relationships within a team should include recognition of each team member and their role and responsibility. Good communication in a team helps members feel that they are listened to and valued, and members should feel able to respectfully discuss and resolve issues within the group (Maryniak 2019).

Standardized Communication

Standardized communication is essential in all aspects of healthcare. Effective communication between the interdisciplinary team and patients and families promote quality and safety. There are many formats for use in healthcare, whether it is for bedside reports or discussing care with other team members, such as a provider. The most common one used is the SBAR, which stands for *S*ituation, *B*ackground, *A*ssessment, and *R*ecommendations. An explanation of the SBAR components are:

- Situation: This is a brief description of what is happening with the patient. This should include the current assessment and vital signs.
- Background: This includes the pertinent history of this patient, as it relates to the problem. This may contain diagnosis, medications, laboratory values, interventions.
- Assessment: This is the assessment of the situation. Describe what the problem is at this time.
- Recommendations: This is any specific request about what the patient needs. Or, during report, this component may be the recommendation of what the patient needs.
    (AHRQ n.d.)

Another useful tool for standardized communication is the I-PASS, which stands for *I*llness severity, *P*atient summary, *A*ction list, *S*ituation awareness, and *S*ynthesis by receiver. Components of the I-PASS are:

- Illness severity: This is a description of how ill the patient is. This may also include code status.
- Patient summary: This is a brief patient overview, including pertinent information such as allergies, weight, hospital course, systems review (if concerns), and any pertinent history.
- Action list: This includes tasks that are pending, such as laboratory results, procedures, and medications.

- Situation awareness: This gives specific information about interventions or what may potentially go wrong. This will help the other person anticipate problems, and be prepared.
- Synthesis by receiver: This allows for questions and clarifications, to ensure that information was received and understood.
    (Blazin et al. 2020)

Strategies Specific to Infection Prevention

Nurses should be aware of the strategies to prevent contamination, particularly working with neonatal patients. This includes avoiding touching hands to face, and limiting touch of potentially contaminated surfaces. Standard precautions should be used judiciously with all patients, regardless of the level of isolation required (CDC 2017). Hand hygiene should be performed frequently and efficiently. Times identified when hand hygiene should be performed include before entering a patient area, before touching a patient, prior to any aseptic procedures, after exposure to blood or body fluids, following touching a patient, after touching the patient environment, and after leaving the patient area. Gloves should also be replaced when heavily soiled or torn (CDC n.d.). A commonly associated contributing cause to outbreaks of hospital-associated infections such as C. diff or MDROs is carrying organisms by the hands of nurses and other healthcare professionals (CDC 2019).

Steps for hand washing are:

1. Wet hands with clean, running water (warm or cold), turn off the tap, and apply soap.
2. Lather hands by rubbing them together with the soap. Lather the backs of the hands, between the fingers, and under the nails.
3. Scrub hands for at least 20 seconds. Need a timer? Hum the "Happy Birthday" song from beginning to end twice.
4. Rinse hands well under clean, running water.
5. Dry hands using a clean towel or air dry them.
    (see Fig. 6.1)

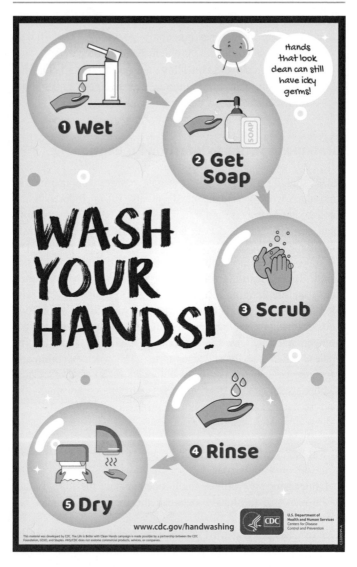

Fig. 6.1 Hand washing graphic. Materials developed by CDC. https://www. cdc.gov/handwashing/pdf/wash-your-hands-poster-english2020-p.pdf.Reference to specific commercial products, manufacturers, companies, or trademarks does not constitute its endorsement or recommendation by the US Government, Department of Health and Human Services, or Centers for Disease Control and Prevention

Steps for hand hygiene using alcohol-based hand rub (ABHR) are:

1. Apply the gel product to the palm of one hand (read the label to learn the correct amount).
2. Rub hands together.
3. Rub the gel over all the surfaces of hands and fingers until hands are dry. This should take around 20 seconds.
    (see Fig. 6.2)

Understanding the PPE requirements for isolation and associated precautions is crucial. This includes communication and appropriate use of PPE in all areas of healthcare (CDC 2019).

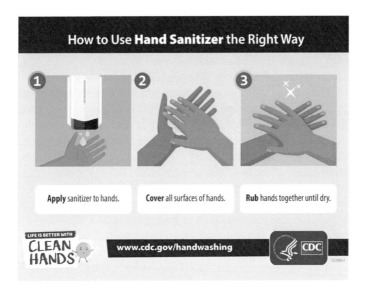

Fig. 6.2 Hand hygiene with ABHR graphic. Materials developed by CDC. https://www.cdc.gov/handwashing/pdf/326806-A_Hand-Sanitizer-SignageSticker-Update-final2_11x8.5in_printonly.pdf. Reference to specific commercial products, manufacturers, companies, or trademarks does not constitute its endorsement or recommendation by the US Government, Department of Health and Human Services, or Centers for Disease Control and Prevention

Approaches for Preventing CLABSIs

The best evidence for preventing CLABSIs include the use of bundles for both insertion and maintenance of central lines. For insertion, strategies include choosing the most appropriate insertion site based on the patient's needs, such as an umbilical venous catheter (UVC), tunneled catheter, or peripherally inserted central catheter (PICC). Hand hygiene and aseptic technique adherence is important prior to insertion. Maximal sterile barriers are required for line insertion. The central line insertion site should be prepared with chlorhexidine and alcohol solution when appropriate for gestational age and skin maturity. Closed systems should be used, with standard precautions used when accessing the devices. Prefilled syringes should be used for flushes, and central line antimicrobial locks may be considered (CDC 2021).

Effective hand hygiene and aseptic technique is also required for central line maintenance. Use of daily bathing with a chlorhexidine solution may be considered when appropriate. Minimizing access to central line hubs is needed. Prior to accessing a port of the central line, vigorous scrubbing of the hub with an appropriate antiseptic (chlorhexidine, iodine, or 70% alcohol) is required. Access to devices is through sterile devices only. Gauze dressings should be changed at least every 48 h, and semipermeable dressings ought to be changed every 7 days. Dressings should also be immediately changed when soiled or loose. IV continuous administration sets should not be changed more frequently than every 96 h, and at least every 7 days. Tubing for blood, blood products, or lipid administration require changing every 24 h. The need for continuing a central line is to be assessed daily, and lines should be immediately removed when no longer required. Umbilical lines should be removed within 7 days (CDC 2021).

Best Practices for Avoiding UTIs

UTIs commonly occur with neonatal patients, and there are many risk factors that cannot be controlled. There are some strategies to help prevent UTIs. Maintaining adequate fluids is one strategy.

Hygiene practices are also essential, including staff performing hand hygiene and using gloves when handling. Frequent diaper changes are needed when wet or soiled. Female patients should be cleaned from front to back, and male patients should have good cleaning of the penis. Using catheters for specimen collection is discouraged with neonates. A urine bag or bladder tap should be used to collect urine (Lai et al. 2018).

Preventing Ventilator-Associated Pneumonia

Ventilator bundles are designed to prevent VAP, but the main initiative against preventing any VAE is to minimize the time the patient is on the ventilator. Strategies include using alternatives to intubation, assessing the need for ventilation daily, and weaning off the ventilator as soon as possible. Weaning from sedation is also important, and use of spontaneous awakening with breathing trials is indicated. Prevention also includes hand hygiene, suctioning only as needed, and use of histamine 2 receptor antagonists or antacids. Oral antimicrobials may be used along with the use of probiotics. Other strategies include providing good oral care frequently with an antiseptic solution. Maintaining elevation of the head of the bed, when appropriate, can prevent aspiration. Use of low tidal volumes and conservative fluid management are also good approaches (Klompas 2019).

Strategies for Preventing Pressure Injuries

Pressure injuries, also known as bedsores, pressure ulcers, or decubitus ulcers, is damage that occurs to the skin and soft tissues. Prolonged pressure, friction, shear, and poor nutritional status can predispose patients to developing pressure injuries. Pressure injuries may or may not be associated with pain. Neonatal patients are at risk for pressure injuries due to immature skin, disease processes, compromised circulation, procedures and surgery, prolonged time in bed, incontinence, medical devices, and pressure on bony prominences (Haesler 2019).

Performing comprehensive skin assessments is essential to identify patients at risk for pressure injury, followed by implementing individualized prevention plans. Standardized risk assessment tools should be used, and the skin should be assessed frequently. The entire skin from head to toe should be examined for abnormalities and injury. This requires visualization under clothes with particular focus on body prominences, and under medical devices (Broom et al. 2019; Haesler 2019).

The skin should be compared symmetrically, noting any differences in skin color, temperature, or areas that do not blanch. Moisture, skin turgor, and skin integrity should be assessed. If wounds or discoloration is noted, this should be documented and photographed (Maryniak 2021).

Staff knowledge of the potential for skin damage and gentle handling is essential for the prevention of skin injury. Staff nails should be short and gloves used with handling. Equipment and supplies can create injury, including the use of adhesives. Minimizing use of equipment to essentials, nominal use of adhesives, removal of any additional supplies within the bed, appropriate cleaning of the neonate, and frequent positioning with developmental support are also needed (Broom et al. 2019).

Prevention of Intraventricular Hemorrhage

Prevention of IVH, especially with VLBW and ELBW neonates is vital, starting before and at delivery. Studies show that antenatal steroids can decrease chance of respiratory distress, which may lower incidence of IVH. Delayed cord clamping, when appropriate, and prompt resuscitation are other strategies to decrease the risk of IVH. It is also important to avoid hemodynamic instability which occurs with hypotension and hypertension. Fluids should be managed and bolus fluids must be avoided when possible. Metabolic homeostasis is needed, which includes avoiding hyperosmolality, hyperglycemia, hypoglycemia, acidosis, and alkalosis. Positioning and developmental care strategies are also essential (Als and McAnulty 2015; Gardner et al. 2020).

Strategies for Preventing Medication Errors

When reviewing strategies to prevent medication errors, there are those at a system level to consider. The National Patient Safety Goals, developed by the Joint Commission, are used as standards for patient safety at organizations throughout the United States. The goals are developed around areas that can be problems in healthcare and are a focus of safety. The 2022 goals include correct patient identification and safe medication use. Other safety goals focus on improving interdisciplinary clinical communication, reducing patient harm associated with clinical alarms, reducing risks of hospital-acquired infections, and identifying patient safety risks (The Joint Commission 2021b).

There are multiple strategies at the system level to help decrease the chance for medication errors, which should be incorporated in organizational processes. The use of two patient identifiers, such as name and date of birth, must be used with medication administration. All medications should be labeled, such as those in syringes or other containers. Anticoagulants, as blood thinners, put patients at higher risk for complications. Extra care and assessment should be practiced with these patients. Maintaining medication reconciliation is important throughout the patient's continuum, including transition from hospital to home, and with every outpatient visit (Maryniak 2018).

Another important focus for system improvement is policies and procedures, such as those involving medication administration. These should be developed based on evidence, and must meet regulatory and accreditation standards. Multidisciplinary team members provide key stakeholders who are involved in medication administration. Shared governance is effective by adding frontline staff who can add valuable insight into policies. Staff buy-in is also improved when they are part of the process, including policy development. Policies differ from guidelines in that they must be followed. Education about policies includes this fact, and staff need to be held accountable for following policies. Organizations should clearly define reporting processes for medication errors. This may include verbal reporting, such as to a provider, and written or electronic reporting processes. Policies for security and access regarding medications should also be created for facilities. This includes those requirements for secured location of medication, and which employees are able to access medications (such as licensed personnel). Medication administration policies may also include the use of technology such as bar-coded medication administration, computerized provider order entry, and smart IV pumps (Maryniak 2018).

Other policy and procedure considerations include safety standards. Organizations should define unacceptable abbreviations. The Joint Commission (2021a) has a list of unacceptable abbreviations, and the Institute for Safe Medication Practices (ISMP) also has extended list of abbreviations, symbols, and other written information which can potentially cause medical errors (ISMP 2021). Unacceptable abbreviations must be defined within a facility. Reference lists are available through the Joint Commission and the Institute for Safe Medication Practices. Examples of unacceptable abbreviations include:

- Avoiding "u" and spelling out "units."
- Avoiding "IU" and spelling out "international units."
- Writing out "daily" and "every other day" rather than using "qd," and "qod."
- Not using trailing 0 after a decimal point.
- Using 0 before a decimal point.
- Writing out morphine sulfate or magnesium sulfate rather than abbreviating with "ms."
- Using "mL" rather than cc.
- Writing out "discharge" or "discontinue" rather than "d/c" abbreviation.
    (ISMP 2021; The Joint Commission 2021a)

High-risk medications need to be defined within the organization, and documentation of practices related to high-risk medication is required. Strategies to decrease risk of medication errors with high-risk medications (ISMP 2018) include:

- Standardization of ordering, storage, preparation, and administration of these medications.
- Improved access to information about these drugs.
- Access to high-alert medications should be limited.
- Supplementary labels and automated alerts can be used.
- Use of redundancies, such as independent double checks.

The ISMP (2018) also has a list of recommended high-risk medications, identified as those which can cause significant patient harm. These include classes of:

- Adrenergic agonists, IV (e.g., epinephrine, phenylephrine, and norepinephrine).
- Adrenergic antagonists, IV (e.g., propranolol, metoprolol, and labetalol).
- Anesthetic agents, general, inhaled, and IV (e.g., propofol and ketamine).
- Antiarrhythmics, IV (e.g., lidocaine and amiodarone).
- Antithrombotic agents, including anticoagulants (e.g., warfarin, low molecular weight heparin, and unfractionated heparin); direct oral anticoagulants and factor Xa inhibitors (e.g., dabigatran, rivaroxaban, apixaban, edoxaban, betrixaban, and fondaparinux); direct thrombin inhibitors (e.g., argatroban, bivalirudin, and dabigatran); glycoprotein IIb/IIIa inhibitors (e.g., eptifibatide); and thrombolytics (e.g., alteplase, reteplase, tenecteplase).
- Cardioplegic solutions.
- Chemotherapeutic agents, both parenteral and oral.
- Dextrose, hypertonic, 20% or greater.
- Dialysis solutions, both peritoneal and hemodialysis.
- Epidural and intrathecal medications.
- Inotropic medications, IV (e.g., digoxin and milrinone).
- Insulin, subcutaneous and IV.
- Liposomal forms of drugs (e.g., liposomal amphotericin B) and conventional counterparts (e.g., amphotericin B desoxycholate).

- Moderate sedation agents, IV (e.g., dexmedetomidine, midazolam, and lorazepam).
- Moderate and minimal sedation agents, oral, for children (e.g., chloral hydrate, midazolam, and ketamine [using the parenteral form]).
- Opioids, including IV; oral (including liquid concentrates, immediate- and sustained-released formulations); transdermal.
- Neuromuscular blocking agents (e.g., succinylcholine, rocuronium, and vecuronium).
- Parenteral nutrition preparations.
- Sodium chloride for injection, hypertonic, greater than 0.9% concentration.
- Sterile water for injection, inhalation, and irrigation (excluding pour bottles) in containers of 100 mL or more.
- Sulfonylurea hypoglycemics, oral (e.g., chlorpropamide, glimepiride, glyburide, glipizide, and tolbutamide).

Specific medications identified as high-risk are:

- Epinephrine, IM, subcutaneous.
- Epoprostenol (e.g., Flolan), IV.
- Insulin U-500 (special emphasis*) (*All forms of insulin, subcutaneous and IV, are considered a class of high-alert medications. Insulin U-500 has been singled out for special emphasis to bring attention to the need for distinct strategies to prevent the types of errors that occur with this concentrated form of insulin).
- Magnesium sulfate injection.
- Methotrexate, oral, non-oncologic use.
- Nitroprusside sodium for injection.
- Opium tincture.
- Oxytocin, IV.
- Potassium chloride for injection concentrate.
- Potassium phosphates injection.
- Promethazine injection.
- Vasopressin, IV, and intraosseous.

Another system consideration for decreasing medication errors is staff resources. Access to expert human resources on medications is needed, such as pharmacists. Medication supplies can be immediately available through unit stock or medication storage, such as electronic dispensaries. Staff need access to medication information, through either a current version of pharmacology textbooks or electronic access, such as online databases or apps. Equipment needed for medication administration should be working and accessible. Examples include IV or syringe pumps, syringes and other supplies, and bar-coded medication technology (Maryniak, 2016 and 2018).

Education, training, the work environment and culture are other system considerations. Both education and experiences help to increase familiarity with commonly used medications. Didactic education for nurses is one strategy, such as inclusion in new graduate nurse residency programs. Clinical experiences include preceptorships with skilled staff to assist knowledge attainment. Work confidence through orientation to the environment can also assist. This can improve time management and decrease stress levels.

Appropriate staffing and workload are common struggles in organizations. Many organizations use ratio-based nursing, which does not consider patient acuity or level of skill of staff. Nurses who are in orientation or preceptorship should not be given full assignments until appropriate. The skill mix needs to consider licensed and unlicensed personnel. Additionally, staffing should consider how many experienced and inexperienced nurses are working during a shift.

Physical environments can impact staff stress and well-being. These can also create distractions from the environment itself. Distractions and interruptions, as commonly identified contributors to errors, must be minimized. Some strategies include use of safe zones that are physically identified in medication rooms or around automated medication dispensaries. Other indicators to limit distractions are the use of tags to identify when a nurse is administering medications. Staff should also be empowered to safely state that he or she must focus on medication administration.

Supervision is a consideration for newer nurses, in particular, when they are learning skills around medication administration. Supportive work environments are those where nurses feel empowered, and participate in shared governance. Teamwork is important to help one another learn and grow, and meet the needs of patients and families. Instituting a just culture is also essential. Visible, supportive leaders who have good relationships with staff create a positive work environment. There must be trust between staff and leaders, which increases an effective culture. Fear or distrust decreases the chance that errors are effectively reported, and therefore processes are not evaluated (Maryniak 2018; Rodziewicz et al. 2021).

System considerations about the use of technology are also needed. As we grow in the use of technology in healthcare, it is important to understand that it is an additional tool to assist staff, but cannot replace critical thinking. Nurses are the last stop to safety with medication administration, and so complacency with technology can be dangerous. Bar-coded medication administration is an important strategy for medication safety. However, not all errors are caught with this technology. For example, if a nurse is to administer a partial dose, it is up to that nurse to appropriately administer the correct dose, like insulin. Additionally, the technology will not necessarily identify when a medication should not be given (such as holding a beta blocker if heart rate or blood pressure is outside parameters). Smart IV pumps are programmed with drug libraries as well as dose reduction systems (which assist with preventing inadvertent high doses). Nurse diligence can assist in identifying and verifying dosages. In one case, new IV pumps were programmed for an incorrect concentration of medication in one facility. A nurse was verifying calculations and caught the error quickly. As a result of her diligence, all of the pumps at the facility were immediately reprogrammed with the right medication concentration (Maryniak 2018).

Just as personal health and stress are correlated with medication errors, personal wellness is associated with better outcomes, and reduced chance for errors. Staff need to ensure that they are getting adequate rest at home and taking breaks at work. It is also important not only to identify areas of stress but also to address the stress, such as the use of coping mechanisms. Staff also need to stay home from work if ill (Rodziewicz et al. 2021).

Nurses must follow the rights of medication administration each and every time. The five basic rights of medication administration are right patient, drug, time, dose, and route. Throughout the years, additional rights have been discussed, up to 12 rights in total, such as right reason, education, documentation, right to refusal, and expiration date. However, the five basic rights are consistently recommended. Nurses are also accountable for following policies and procedures. If there is unfamiliarity with policies, then referring to them should be done until familiar. Nurses should never give any medication without knowing the reason, possible side effects, interactions, safe dose range, monitoring, etc. (Rodziewicz et al. 2021).

Nurses as advocates can assist the family with effective teaching, and encourage them to speak up if there are any concerns or if they do not understand something. Nurses must also listen to concerns. For example, if a family states "Oh, the doctor said he was going to stop giving my baby that medication," then the nurse should verify before either administering or holding a medication. Promoting self-wellness and a supportive work culture assists everyone, including patients and families (Maryniak 2018).

Using a Daily Management System

As discussed in Chap. 5, the use of a daily management system (DMS) can increase awareness, improve communication, foster transparency, help reduce errors, and improve safety. Daily management allows staff doing the work and leaders at all levels of the organization to clearly visualize whether the performance is on track (no variations) or has deviated from target condition(s). Some key points about DMS are:

- A DMS helps to rapidly identify deviation and correct the problem by bringing attention to the problem and quickly addressing the cause.

- Everyone has equal responsibility for taking necessary actions to quickly correct the problem or escalate as needed.
- Old school of thought brought attention to the problem after the fact making it difficult to find causation and fix; DMS brings immediate attention with expectation to address causation or escalate barriers as needed.

One example is the focus on reducing CLABSIs. A system goal would be zero harm, with a facility goal of reducing CLABSI events. The department's goal would then be decreasing the indwelling central line catheter days (see Fig. 6.3).

The dwell time has the highest impact on developing CLABSIs—each day increases the chance of infection. Therefore, if the dwell time can be reduced then CLABSIs can also be decreased.

The room number of patients with central lines would be placed on the DMS board, and these patients would be prioritized in leader and interdisciplinary rounding to ensure they meet the criteria for the line or it is removed. The same principle would be used for hospital-acquired pressure injuries (HAPIs) as well (see Fig. 6.4).

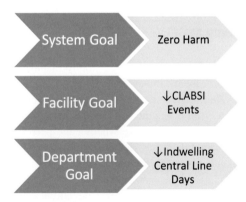

Fig. 6.3 Alignment of goals

Outcome metric	# since last huddle	Days since last incidence	Process metric today	Comments
Central lines	5	N/A	N/A	Beds 1, 14, 16, 22, 24
CLABSI	0	250	100%	Bundle compliance goal 95%
Skin injury	0	22	100%	
Ventilators	6	N/A	N/A	Beds 1, 2, 14, 16, 22, 24
VAP	0	165	95%	Bundle compliance goal 95%
Hand hygiene	N/A	N/A	75%	Bundle compliance goal 95%

Fig. 6.4 Example of process monitoring on DMS board

It is important to prioritize rounding and monitoring to aid in reduction of harmful events. Whenever a patient has a device, they should be monitored closely to ensure the device is needed, and if so, the correct processes involved with care of the device are strictly adhered to. The only way to effectively monitor this is by making it a priority.

Best Practices for Developmental Care

Environmental strategies can promote the growth and development of the neonate and reduce stress. Approaches are to reduce noise, have soft lighting, cluster patient care, limit bedside activity, and have visual surroundings that are soothing. Patients can also be shielded from sound and light when incubators are used. The use of soft music has also been known to be helpful, but it is important to monitor the neonate's reaction. Family and staff should be provided education on the importance of creating and maintaining a calming environment that does not disrupt sleep. It should also be noted that the actions of staff at the bedside set an example for the family (Als and McAnulty 2015; Gardner et al. 2020).

The primary team and family should develop care plans together that meet the medical and developmental needs of the neonate, with the goal to maximize rest, minimize stress, and optimize healing and growth. Positioning should focus on providing comfort and ability for self-regulation. The use of nesting materials, sheepskin, or blanket rolls will help the neonate maintain its position. Swaddling is appropriate as long as there is the ability for the neonate's hands to go to the face for self-comfort. Hands-on containment during procedures is essential, and families or ancillary staff can assist. Parental skin-to-skin contact (kangaroo care) provides comfort, promotes bonding, and provides positive tactile and olfactory experiences (Als and McAnulty 2015; Gardner et al. 2020).

Non-pharmacological interventions to relieve discomfort and pain include swaddling, giving pacifiers, holding, rocking, and giving oral sucrose solution, if not contraindicated. Pharmacological interventions for pain should also be utilized, especially while on a ventilator or with other invasive procedures (Als and McAnulty 2015; Gardner et al. 2020).

There are also developmentally appropriate feeding strategies. When preparing the neonate and mother to breastfeed, kangaroo care is an excellent approach. Premature neonates should be put to breast as soon as they are stable because although they may not feed, they can nuzzle with their mother and the neonate will benefit from closeness. Gavage feedings can be improved by wrapping and holding the neonates, with a pacifier for nonnutritive sucking. If bottle feeding, swaddling the neonate and lying on their side to feed can decrease stress. Another consideration with bottle feeding is to choose the appropriate nipple flow rate for the level of feeding competency (Als and McAnulty 2015; Gardner et al. 2020).

References

Als H, McAnulty G (2015) Developmental care guidelines for use in the newborn intensive care unit (NICU). NIDCAP Federation International Web site http://www.inha.ie/wp-content/uploads/2015/07/INHA_Developmental_Care_Guidelines.pdf

Agency for Healthcare Research and Quality (AHRQ) (n.d.) Nurse bedside shift report: Implementation handbook. https://www.ahrq.gov/sites/default/files/wysiwyg/professionals/systems/hospital/engagingfamilies/strategy3/Strat3_Implement_Hndbook_508.pdf

Blazin LJ, Sitthi-Amorn J, Hoffman JM, Burlison JD (2020) Improving patient handoffs and transitions through adaptation and implementation of I-PASS across multiple handoff settings. Pediatric Quality & Safety 5(4):e323

Broom M, Dunk A, Mohamed E, A. (2019) Predicting neonatal skin injury: the first step to reducing skin injuries in neonates. Health Service Insights 14:12

Centers for Disease Control & Prevention (n.d.) Sequence for putting on personal protective equipment (PPE). https://www.cdc.gov/hai/pdfs/ppe/ppe-sequence.pdf

Centers for Disease Control & Prevention (2017) Management of multidrug-resistant organisms in healthcare settings, 2006 (updated 2017). https://www.cdc.gov/infectioncontrol/pdf/guidelines/mdro-guidelines.pdf

Centers for Disease Control & Prevention (2019) 2007 guideline for isolation precautions: preventing transmission of infectious agents in healthcare settings (updated 2019). https://www.cdc.gov/infectioncontrol/pdf/guidelines/isolation-guidelines-H.pdf

Centers for Disease Control & Prevention (2021) NICU: CLABSI guidelines. https://www.cdc.gov/infectioncontrol/guidelines/nicu-clabsi/index.html

Cham P, Ellsworth L, Gisondo C, Lawrence C, Weiner G (2021) An analysis of neonatal intensive care daily rounds in a level IV unit. Pediatrics 147(3_MeetingAbstract):420–421

Dorvil B (2018) The secrets to successful nurse bedside shift report implementation and sustainability. Nurs Manag 49(6):20–25

Gardner SL, Carter BS, Enzman-Hines M, Niermeyer S (2020) Merenstein & Gardner's handbook of neonatal intensive care, 9th edn. Mosby Elsevier

Haesler E (2019) Prevention and treatment of pressure ulcers/injuries: the international guideline 2019. Cambridge Media

Institute for Safe Medication Practices (2018) High alert medications in acute care settings. https://www.ismp.org/recommendations/high-alert-medications-acute-list

Institute for Safe Medication Practices (2021) ISMP's list of error-prone abbreviations, symbols, and dose designations. https://www.ismp.org/Tools/errorproneabbreviations.pdf

Klompas M (2019) Ventilator-associated events: what they are and what they are not. Respir Care, 64(8), 953–961

Lai A, Rove K, Amin S, Vricella G, Coplen D (2018) Diagnosis and management of urinary tract infections in premature and term infants. NeoReviews 19(6):e337–e348

Maryniak K (2016) How to avoid medication errors in nursing. https://www.rn.com/nursing-news/nurses-role-in-medication-error-prevention/

Maryniak K (2018) Medication errors: best practices for prevention (webinar). Lorman

Maryniak K (2019) Professional nursing practice in the United States: an overview for international nurses, and those along the continuum from new graduates to experienced nurses

Maryniak K (2021) Documentation for nurses, 4th edn. Elite Healthcare

Rodziewicz TL, Houseman B, Hipskind JE (2021) Medical error reduction and prevention. In StatPearls. StatPearls Publishing. https://pubmed.ncbi.nlm.nih.gov/29763131/

Shivananda S, Osiovich H, de Salaberry J, Hait V, Gautham K (2022) Improving efficiency of multidisciplinary bedside rounds in the NICU: a single Centre QI project. Pediatric Quality & Safety 7(1):e511

The Joint Commission (2021a) Facts about the official "Do Not Use" list of abbreviations. https://www.jointcommission.org/facts_about_do_not_use_list/

The Joint Commission (2021b) 2022 hospital national patient safety goals. https://www.jointcommission.org/standards/national-patient-safety-goals/hospital-national-patient-safety-goals/

Case Studies

7

Case Study #1

Baby Marie was born at 32 weeks gestation and was admitted to the open-concept neonatal intensive care unit. She had TTNB when born but recovered well, and at 10 days of age was on room air, and feeding and growing. On night shift, the nurse noted that Marie had redness in both eyes. It also appeared that Marie's eyes were watery and irritating to her.

Two days later, the patient in the next bed, baby William, was also noted to have watery, red eyes. William was a 5-day-old male, born at 30 weeks gestation, on high-flow nasal cannula and on an open warmer. The same day that William began with symptoms, another patient in the unit, baby Dot, developed the same symptoms. Dot was a 3-day-old female, born at 34 weeks, who was under phototherapy.

The charge nurse identified the trend with the patient's signs and symptoms and called the infection preventionist. All three patients were placed in contact plus standard precautions. The provider took cultures from the three patients, which were positive for bacterial conjunctivitis.

K. Maryniak, *Controlling and Preventing Errors and Pitfalls in Neonatal Care Delivery*, https://doi.org/10.1007/978-3-031-25710-0_7

The nursing manager, risk manager, and infection preventionist determined that a root cause analysis would be warranted in this situation. They invited nurses, providers, and respiratory therapists to the RCA.

• In reviewing the spread of conjunctivitis among the patients, why could this happen?

The group participating in the RCA, using the five whys, determined the contributing factors involved (see Fig. 7.1).

The RCA group discussed that there were appropriate processes in place, through policies and procedures, about hand hygiene and environmental cleaning. They also identified that there were appropriate equipment and supplies available for hand hygiene and environmental cleaning. The staff determined that the most likely cause of the cases of conjunctivitis was spread through staff. This finding aligns with statements from the CDC, that outbreaks often occur from a failure to uphold infection prevention and control practices (CDC 2021). The group admitted that there were missed opportunities for both hand hygiene and environmental cleaning among staff, including themselves. Examples included not changing gloves and performing hand hygiene when working from dirty to clean, not always performing hand hygiene at each opportunity (especially if there was a sense of urgency between patients), and not cleaning the environment (such as counters or bedside tables) with every opportunity. These behaviors were identified as at-risk, using a just culture process. Contributing factors also included the need to reinforce infection prevention practices, hold staff accountable for these practices, and communicate results from infection prevention audits (see Fig. 7.2).

Findings from the RCA were shared with leadership, and a corrective action plan was created to be implemented within the department (see Fig. 7.3).

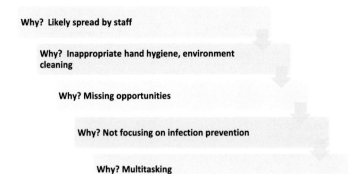

Fig. 7.1 Five whys for RCA in case study one

Category	Contributing Factors
People	Missing opportunities for hand hygiene and environmental cleaning; not focusing
Processes	Processes for hand hygiene and cleaning were in place
Equipment, supplies	Equipment and supplies were available
Culture	Need reinforcement of accountability for hand hygiene, appropriate use of PPE, environmental cleaning
Communication	Communication of hand hygiene audits were not done with staff
Staffing, training	Need to reinforce hand hygiene, PPE, and environmental cleaning practices

Fig. 7.2 Contributing factors of RCA for case study one

Corrective Action	Measure of Success	Responsible Party	Due to Review
Re-educate staff on infection prevention measures, including reinforcing appropriate hand hygiene, use of PPE, and environmental cleaning practices	Staff will successfully pass post-test with a minimum of 80%	Clinical Education	One month
Hand hygiene audits will be performed and results shared with staff	Audits will show 95% compliance with hand hygiene 100% of results will be posted on DMS board and reviewed with all staff	Infection Prevention	Monthly
Managers will reinforce accountability for infection prevention practices, including hand hygiene, appropriate use of PPE, environmental cleaning with staff	Infection prevention practices will be documented in staff performance reviews Progressive discipline, if warranted based on just culture, will occur for not following infection prevention practices	Managers	Ongoing

Fig. 7.3 Corrective action plan for case study one

Case Study #2

A nurse leader, Nicole, was rounding on the unit and saw a new nurse Stephanie (who was just off orientation) performing a central line tubing change on her own. The policy and procedure in the level III NICU were to have two staff at the bedside to perform sterile procedures, including changing the tubing with central lines. Nicole also noted that Stephanie contaminated the new line as she was preparing to hook it up.

Nicole joined Stephanie at the bedside and stopped the procedure, and had her start over, with Nicole assisting. Nicole walked Stephanie through the procedure and helped her maintain sterility throughout.

After completion of the procedure, Nicole had a private conversation with Stephanie and asked her what education she had been given for performing central line changes. Stephanie stated she had only participated in a line change once, and tried to follow what her preceptor was doing. She also said that she only had one opportunity to practice sterile technique in a skills lab during her nursing school. Stephanie was not aware that she had broken sterile technique, or that two people were needed for the procedure. Nicole identified that this was human error, and that Stephanie needed more education and reinforcement. Nicole spoke with Stephanie about the importance of following the policy and procedure, and to have knowledge of sterile techniques.

Nicole also realized that Stephanie's preceptor, Rick, might need more information, and so she spoke with him. Nicole learned that Rick had very little experience with central line changes, since he had just transferred from a lower level of neonatal care, where central lines were used infrequently. Rick stated that his orientation felt rushed, and there were learning opportunities for him as well.

Nicole worked with the educator, and they revised the orientation for new nurses to include simulation with sterile technique. Preceptor education was also revised based on feedback. Communications with staff were done, reminding them of where policies and procedures were located. Additionally, competencies were developed for sterile technique and central line tubing changes. Monthly audits were instituted following education, which showed an increase in compliance with sterile technique and central line maintenance, including tubing changes.

Reference

Centers for Disease Control and Prevention (CDC) (2021) Outbreak investigations in healthcare settings. https://www.cdc.gov/hai/outbreaks/index.html

Recommendations for Further Study

8

It has been noted that there are studies that examine various errors in nursing and in healthcare. The frequency of errors directly related to neonatal patients is not commonly seen in the literature. For example, there are many studies that examine adult hospital-acquired conditions such as CLABSI, CAUTI, and VAP, but not as many look specifically at conditions in the neonatal population. Additionally, studies regarding errors have mainly focused on medication errors. There are opportunities in the literature to further delve into neonatal-specific conditions and nursing practices. This should be done in all neonatal settings, including different levels of neonatal intensive care, nursery settings, pediatric and labor and delivery settings. Errors in neonatal ambulatory settings such as clinics or follow-up programs in the home can also be examined.

Neonatal patients are very specialized, and the level of acuity can vary from healthy to acutely ill. More examination of environmental contributing factors that can lead to errors may be warranted. The work environment, stress, additional time constraints, and current changes in the workforce can increase the risk of errors with neonatal patients. There may also be additional stacking in the minds of nurses caring for these patients, which can also lead to errors. There are also opportunities to further delve into specific systems and personal contributing factors for errors. Examining organizational traits, including staffing practices, use

K. Maryniak, *Controlling and Preventing Errors and Pitfalls in Neonatal Care Delivery*, https://doi.org/10.1007/978-3-031-25710-0_8

of skill mix, and incorporation of best practices into policies and procedures compared with error rates can provide valuable information. It is important to examine personal considerations that may correlate with error rates, including years of experience, education, certification, and leader qualities.

Examining the personal effects of errors from the perspective of the family, and nurse is also required. Both quantitative and qualitative studies would add significance to this topic.

Summary

Caring for neonatal patients requires complex nursing care. Baseline knowledge about common neonatal conditions is essential for nursing staff. There are errors that can occur related to nursing care, such as inappropriate or omitted hand hygiene, medication errors, or hospital-acquired conditions. Errors with a neonate can create lifelong consequences.

There are multiple factors that can contribute to nursing errors, both at system and personal levels. Together, organizations, leaders, and staff are accountable for ensuring there are appropriate processes for reducing the risk of errors. Diligence, communication, and a constant focus on safety are required.

Potential or actual errors can create a near-miss situation or one with actual harm. Consequences of nursing errors can be detrimental to many people, not just the patient. Patients, families, and healthcare professionals can all be affected by errors.

Effective systems must be in place to properly monitor for and detect nursing errors. These systems should be beneficial to all key stakeholders, and add value to processes. Use of a just culture in an organization is necessary for reporting, monitoring, and creating change.

Nurses should keep up to date with evidence-based practices. The use of bundles, developmental care considerations, and interdisciplinary rounding are all examples. As healthcare continues to evolve and research is done, changes in practice will continue to focus on what is learned to provide the best quality care to patients.

© The Editor(s) (if applicable) and The Author(s), under exclusive license to Springer Nature Switzerland AG 2023
K. Maryniak, *Controlling and Preventing Errors and Pitfalls in Neonatal Care Delivery*, https://doi.org/10.1007/978-3-031-25710-0

Printed by Libri Plureos GmbH
in Hamburg, Germany